Community
Health Nursing-I
Record Book
for BSc Nursing Program

Community Health Nursing-I
Record Book

Semester V

for BSc Nursing Program

As per the Revised INC Syllabus

Third Edition

C Manivannan
MSc (N) MPhil (Psy) PhD (N)
Vice Principal and Head
Department of Child Health Nursing
Shri Bharani College of Nursing
Salem, Tamil Nadu, India

T Latha Manivannan
MSc (N) PhD (N)
Vice Principal and Head
Department of Community Health Nursing
Kailash College of Nursing
Salem, Tamil Nadu, India

S Rathamani
MSc (N)
Nursing Officer
Krishnagiri Government Hospital
Salem, Tamil Nadu, India

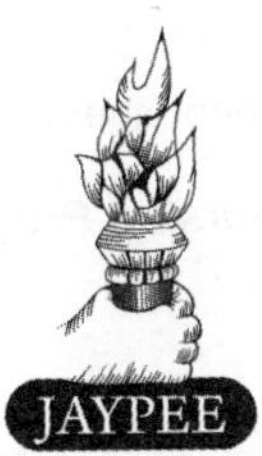

JAYPEE BROTHERS MEDICAL PUBLISHERS
The Health Sciences Publisher
New Delhi | London

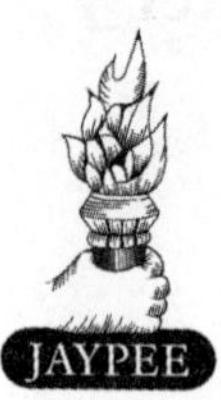

Jaypee Brothers Medical Publishers (P) Ltd

Headquarters
EMCA House, 23/23-B
Ansari Road, Daryaganj
New Delhi 110 002, India
Landline: +91-11-23272143,
+91-11-23272703
+91-11-23282021, +91-11-23245672
e-mail: jaypee@jaypeebrothers.com

Overseas Office
JP Medical Ltd.
83, Victoria Street, London
SW1H 0HW (UK)
Phone: +44-20 3170 8910
e-mail: info@jpmedpub.com

Corporate Office
4838/24, Ansari Road, Daryaganj
New Delhi 110 002, India
Phone: +91-11-43574357
Fax: +91-11-43574314
e-mail: jaypee@jaypeebrothers.com

EU GPSR Authorised Representative
Logos Europe, 9 rue Nicolas Poussin
17000, La Rochelle, France
Phone: +33 (0) 6 67 93 73 78
e-mail: contact@logoseurope.eu

Website: www.jaypeebrothers.com
Website: www.jaypeedigital.com

Inquiries for bulk sales may be solicited at: jaypee@jaypeebrothers.com

Community Health Nursing-I: Record Book for BSc Nursing Program (Semester V)

First Edition: 2014

Second Edition: 2022

Third Edition: **2024**

Reprint: **2026**

ISBN: 978-93-5696-569-0

Printed in India at Purewall Ventures Pvt Ltd

Preface

Community Health Nursing-I Record Book for BSc Nursing Program (Semester V) is prepared according to the requirements of community health nursing-I for BSc Nursing and is aimed to provide a simple and systematic record book on community health nursing for undergraduate students. The BSc Nursing students are guided by their teachers in various aspects to maintain quality and standards for community experience based on the requirements, which were established or maintained for every college of nursing in India.

This record book is updated and based on the Indian Nursing Council (INC) syllabus, including the mid-level health provider (MLHP) program, specifically designed for the BSc Nursing program in community health nursing for 5th semester students. This record book presents the subject in 5th semester procedures with important notes and explanations for community health nursing, which will certainly meet the needs of students.

This book maintains good community experience based on requirements in a standardized format, which minimizes the workload of clinical instructors and students. The students are self-guided with the help of this book during the time of community visit. These formats are standardized and based on community requirement, which can be followed by the students in an easy manner. It also helps the students to maintain all the records of community experience, which will help the clinical instructors to evaluate the student's activity in the community area.

We hope that this book will be an asset in the field of community health nursing.

C Manivannan
T Latha Manivannan
S Rathamani

Acknowledgments

- First of all, we would like to thank the Almighty for giving us the strength, patience, and good health to successfully complete this book.
- We owe our heartiest and greatest thanks to Chairman **Dr S Rajamanickom, MS (Ortho), D Ortho, MAMS (Vienna), MCh (Ortho) Managing Director of Shri Bharani College of Nursing (SBCON), Salem**, and Secretary **Dr Punithavathi, MBBS, DGO, DMRD, SBCON,** for their constant encouragement and support.
- We express our warm gratitude to all our colleagues and friends for their constant encouragement in writing this record book.
- We take this opportunity to express our sincere thanks to our parents, sisters, and brothers for their unselfish love, endless patience, and quiet understanding that allowed us to successfully complete this book.
- We express our warm gratitude to the whole team of M/s Jaypee Brothers Medical Publishers (P) Ltd, New Delhi, India, who helped and guided us—Shri Jitendar P Vij (Group Chairman), Mr Ankit Vij (Managing Director), Mr MS Mani (Group President), Dr Madhu Choudhary (Director–Educational Publishing), Ms Pooja Bhandari [Director–Production (Books and Journals)], Ms Sunita Katla (Executive Assistant to Group Chairman and Publishing Manager), Mr Ajay Kumar Sharma [Deputy General Manager (Books and Journals)], Ms Samina Khan (Executive Assistant to Director–Educational Publishing), Ms Alisha Talwar (Team Lead–Nursing), Mr Rajesh Sharma (Production Coordinator), Ms Seema Dogra (Cover Visualizer), Ms Neha Verma (Graphic Designer–Cover), Mr Anil Singh (Proofreader), Mr Akshay Thakur (DTP Typesetter), Mr Suhel Ahmed (Graphic Designer), and their team members, for all their support while working in this project and making it a success.
- We are sincerely thankful to Mr Kumar C (Sales Executive, Bengaluru Branch), M/s Jaypee Brothers Medical Publishers (P) Ltd, Bengaluru Karnataka, for his wholehearted cooperation.

Community Health Nursing Record Book for
BSc Nursing Program

Name of the Institution   : _______________________________________

(IN BLOCK LETTERS)

Place   : _______________________________________

Name of the Student   : _______________________________________

Register Number   : _______________________________________

Date of Posting (V semester)   : From: _______________ To: _______________

Date of Posting (VII semester)   : From: _______________ To: _______________

Signature of the Student   : _______________________________________

PHOTOGRAPH

Name and Signature of Clinical Instructor
Date:

Name and Signature
Head of Department of Community Health Nursing:
Date:

College Seal

Name and Signature of Internal Examiner
Date:

1.
2.

Name and Signature of External Examiner
Date:

1.
2.

Contents

Introduction—Short Notes on Community Health Nursing During Practice — **1**

Essential Requirements for Community Health Nursing — **17**

1. Orientation — 21
2. Community Assessment — 24
3. Community Survey — 32
4. Household Survey — 40
5. Family Folder — 60
6. Community Field Visits — 85
7. Observation Visit for Nutrition Programme — 92
8. Observational Visits — 143
9. Health Education/Counseling — 155
10. Preparation of Audiovisual Aids — 162
11. Family Care Plan — 176
12. Family Care Study — 212
13. Biomedical Waste Management — 246
14. Records and Reports — 251
15. Notification of Disease — 252
16. Identification of Communicable Diseases and Noncommunicable Diseases — 254
17. Bag Techniques — 261
18. National Health Programmes — 274

GENERAL OBJECTIVES OF COMMUNITY VISIT

Purpose of the Experience

- The students are able to understand the administrative setup and functions of administration in different areas of nursing service such as in the community health nursing setup.
- They are able to identify and analyze problem in administration and suggest possible remedies with the application of problem-solving.
- The students are able to identify and critically analyze the existing problems in administration.

■ COMMUNITY HEALTH NURSING

A field of nursing that is a blend of primary healthcare and nursing practice with public health nursing. The community health nurse conducts a continuing and comprehensive practice that is preventive, curative and rehabilitative. The philosophy of care is based on the belief that care directed to the individual, the family and the group contributes to the healthcare of the population as a whole. The community health nurse is not restricted to the care of a particular age or diagnostic group. Participation of all consumers of healthcare is encouraged in the development of community activities that contributes to the promotion of education and maintenance of good health. These activities require comprehensive health programs that pay special attention to social and ecological influences and specific populations at risk.

■ PURPOSE OF THE FIELD OR COMMUNITY EXPERIENCE

The students understand the administrative setup and functions of administration in different areas of nursing service that is in the community health setup. They can identify and analyze the problems in administration and suggest possible remedies with the application of problem solving.

The students are able to identify and critically analyze the existing problem in administration.

■ METHODS OF STUDY

1. Observation.
2. Questionnaire.
3. Discussion with concerned personnel in each area.
4. Written assignments.
5. Presentation of reports:
   - Describe the community health nursing setup as observed.
   - Students are able to understand and explain:
     - Community health nursing administration organized on healthcare public system, 5 year plan, primary healthcare.
     - Scope of community health nursing (administrative supervisory teaching and research).
     - Functions of public health nurse in homes, clinic, urban and rural, general and special.
     - Health centers: Rural–primary health centers, subcenters.
     - Hospitals industries.
     - Training at community health centers, teaching institutions, school and college of nursing, multipurpose workers' school.
     - Regional family welfare training center.
     - Institute of public health.
     - District public health office—general and family welfare.
     - Health education bureau—central and state.
     - Applied nutrition program.
     - National welfare control and eradication programs—tuberculosis, leprosy, malaria and others.
     - Special projects, WHO, Danida and others, handicapped children.
     - Responsibilities of community health nursing (CHN) in the care of handicapped children.
     - Implication of the aging population in relation to preventive and social medicine problems.
     - Community health and program planning steps.
       » Plan formation
       » Execution

- » Evaluation
- » Health needs and demands
- » Resources
- » Objectives
- » Targets
- » Goals
- » Plans
- ◆ Community organization.
- ◆ Role of community leaders:
  - » Identification and training of community leaders.
  - » Training and supervision of community level workers.

■ TERMINOLOGY

- **Agent:** A biological, physical or chemical entry, capable of causing diseases.
- **Antibody:** A protein substance that produces resistance power, naturally or artificially.
- **Antigen:** It is a foreign substance that induces an immune response in the body.
- **Antiserum:** Serum containing specific antibody.
- **Attack rate:** A measurement of the frequency of new cases.
- **Carrier:** A person/animal who carries the disease agent.
- **Communicable disease:** An illness due to specific infectious agent, which is spread from one person to another person.
- **Endemic:** The condition, which is present within the population.
- **Epidemic:** An outbreak of disease in a community in excess of normal expectation and derived from a common source (e.g., cholera).
- **Fomites:** Inanimate article other than food and water, e.g., pen, pencil and handkerchief, etc.
- **Incubation period:** This is the time interval between entry of disease agent into the body and appearance of the first signs and symptoms of disease.
- **Infection:** The entry and development or multiplication of disease-producing agent in the body of man or animal; may or may not lead to disease.
- **Isolation:** Separation of patient with infectious disease.
- **Noncommunicable disease:** A condition or disease, which is noninfectious and nontransmissible; this is applied in case of anemia and diabetes mellitus.
- **Pandemic:** An epidemic, which spreads from country-to-country or whole world.
- **Pathogenesis:** Ability to cause disease.
- **Sporadic:** The incidence occurring at intervals of single or scattered cases of disease.
- **Vector:** Usually an agent, which transfers infection to person, e.g. anthropoid, insect.
- **Virulent:** Measuring the severity of diseases.
- **Zoonosis:** Disease, which is transmitted from animal to man.

■ PRINCIPLES OF COMMUNITY HEALTH NURSING

- Community health nurse has to provide care based on needs of individuals, families and communities.
- The community health nurse has to achieve the goal by the use of knowledge, and understanding of the objectives and policies of the agency.
- Community health nurse considers the family as fundamental unit for providing preventive, promotive and curative services.
- Respect for the values, customs and beliefs of the clients, contributes to the effectiveness of care to the client. Community health nurse service must be available in a sustainable and affordable manner to all regardless of race, creed, color and socioeconomic status.
- Community health nurse integrates health education and counseling as vital parts of functions. They encourage and support community peoples to improve the health.

- Community health nurse has to improve relationships with the coworkers and members of the health team. This facilities the accomplishments of goals. Each member should be helped to observe how the work benefits the whole enterprise.
- Community health nurse should have periodic and continuing evaluation of work to fulfill and achieve goals and objectives of program. Clients are involved in the appraisal of their health program through consultations, observations and accurate recording.
- Community health nurse should have professional interest; they consider formulating plan of staff development programs to improve the quality service. It is essential to upgrade and maintain sound nursing practices.
- Utilization of indigenous and existing community resources, maximizes the success of the efforts of the community health nurses. The use of local available elements and linkages with existing community resources—both public and private, increase the awareness of what care they need that are entitled.
- Community health nursing program needs active participation of the individual, family and community in planning and making decisions for their healthcare needs to a large extent for its success. Organized community groups are encouraged to participate in the activities that will meet community needs and interests.
- Supervision of nursing services by qualified community health nursing personnel to provide guidance and direction to the work to be done. Potentials of employees for effective and efficient work are developed.
- Accurate recording and reporting serves as the basis for evaluation of the progress of planned programs and activities and acts as a guide for future actions. Maintenance of accurate records is a vital responsibility of community, as these are utilized in studies and researches, and as legal documents.

■ LEVELS OF PREVENTION

The goals of medicine are to promote health for preventing diseases and to restore health when it is impaired.

- Primordial prevention
- Primary prevention
- Secondary prevention
- Tertiary prevention

Primordial Prevention

- Primordial prevention is a new concept, receiving special attention in the prevention of chronic diseases, such as diabetes mellitus, hypertension, etc.
- Since primordial prevention is the pure form of primary prevention, the problems like obesity, hypertension can be prevented.
- Efforts are directed towards discouraging children from adapting harmful life practices. The harmful lifestyle leads to disease by modifying the lifestyles, e.g., smoking, eating pattern.
- Mode of intervention in health education.

Primary Prevention

- Action taken prior to the onset of disease, which removes the possibility of disease that will ever occur.
- Primary prevention signifies intervention in the prepathogens phase.
- Primary prevention includes the concept of positive health that encourages achievement and maintenance of an acceptable level of health that will enable every individual to lead socially and economically protective life.
- The concept of primary prevention is now being applied to the prevention of chronic diseases, such as coronary heart disease, hypertension and cancer, based on elimination or modification of risk factors of disease.

Secondary Prevention

Secondary prevention can be defined as actions, which halts progress of a disease, performed in incipient stage and prevent complication.

Intervention

- Early diagnosis and adequate treatment (screening test)
- By early diagnosis and treatment, secondary prevention attempt to arrest the disease process and restore health by seeking out unrecognized disease, treating it before irreversible pathological changes takes place and reverse communicability of infectious disease.
- Secondary prevention protect others in the community from the infection.
- They provide at once secondary prevention for the infected individuals and primary prevention for their contacts.
- Secondary prevention is largely the domain of clinical medicine.
- The health programs initiated by governments are usually at the level of secondary prevention.
- The drawback of secondary prevention is that the patient has already been subjected to mental anguish, physical and the community to lose a production.
- Secondary prevention is an imperfective tool in the control of transmission of disease.
- Secondary prevention is more expensive and less effective.

Tertiary Prevention

- When the disease process has advantage beyond its early stages.
- Tertiary prevention is still possible if it accomplishes prevention by what might be called tertiary prevention.
- Tertiary prevention significance intervention in the late pathogen phase.
- Tertiary prevention can be defined as all measures available to reduce all limit impairment and disability, minimize suffering caused by existence; departure from good health and promote the patient adjustment to immediate condition, e.g., treatment, even if undertaken late in the natural history of disease, may prevent sequences and limit disability.
- When defect and disability have more or less stabilized producer of its own pattern of disease.
- The term of this will be obvious when compared with the leading causes of death in developed countries.

◼ PROCEDURES DURING HOME VISIT

Bag Technique

- The community bag consists of front pouch, side pouches, lower compartment and upper compartment. Outside pouch consist of handwashing articles, such as soap with soap dish, nail brush, nail cutter and towel.
- The frontside pouch consist of newspaper and physical examination articles, such as scale, fetus scope, stethoscope, inch tape, etc.
- The backside pouch consists of paper bag, hemoglobin estimation scale, pen, paper, diary, etc.
- The lower compartment consist of clean articles, such as kidney tray, spirit lamp, test tube holder, match box, etc.
- The upper compartment consist of sterile articles, such as temperature pack, dressing pack, injection pack, oral medications, injections, solutions, ointment, test tubes, slides, etc.
  - Always keep the bag at the right side.
  - Take the newspaper and spread it, the inner side of the newspaper should face upward.
  - Keep the bag at the comer of the newspaper; the outside pouch should be placed at the backside.
  - First take the handwashing articles from the outside pouch.
  - Take the needed articles from the clean compartment or side pouches.
  - Do handwashing.
  - Take the needed articles from the upper compartment.
  - Close the upper compartment.
  - Do the procedure.
  - Clean the articles.
  - Do handwashing.
  - Replace the sterile articles first, then replace the clean articles and side pouch articles.
  - Replace the handwashing articles.
  - Close the bag.

Temperature Technique

- Open the front pouch, take the handwashing articles.
- Open the side pouch, take the paper bag, diary and pen.
- Open the lower compartment and take the kidney tray.
- Do handwashing.
- Open the sterile compartment and take the temperature pack. It consists of thermometer, cotton balls and cotton pad.
- Close the upper compartment.
- Open the thermometer pack and take the thermometer from the pouch. Take one cotton ball and clean the thermometer from bulb to stem and discard in the paper bag.
- Keep the thermometer under the tongue of the client.
- Wait for 3 minutes and remove the thermometer and take another cotton ball, clean from stem to bulb and discard in the paper bag.
- Read the mercury level and record it in the diary.
- Take the cotton pad, wet it and apply the soap and roll the thermometer and keep it in the kidney tray for 3 minutes.
- After 3 minutes remove the soapy cotton and discard it in the paper bag.
- Wash the thermometer under the running water.
- Take another cotton ball, clean the thermometer from stem to bulb and keep it in the pouch.
- Burn the paper bag.
- Clean the kidney tray.
- Do handwashing.
- Replace the thermometer pouch in the upper compartment.
- Replace the kidney tray in the lower compartment.
- Replace the handwashing articles and close the bag.

Urine Test

- Open the bag and take the handwashing articles.
- Open the side pouch and take pen and diary.
- Open the lower compartment and take the kidney tray, specimen bottle, spirit lamp, match box, test tube holder.
- Do handwashing.
- Open the upper compartment and take test tubes and solutions.
- Close the bag.
- Take the test tube and hold it in test tube holder; pour 5 mL of Benedict's solution and heat it.
- Watch the color change. If it is blue, continue or if any other color change occurs, discard it.
- In 5 mL of Benedict's solution, after the heating, add eight drops of urine and boil it.
- Make it cool and watch the color change:
  - *Blue:* Negative
  - *Green:* 1%
  - *Yellow:* 2%
  - *Orange:* 3%
  - *Brick red:* Above 5%.
- Enter the result.
- Discard the waste.
- Clean the articles.
- Do handwashing.
- Replace the upper compartment articles and replace the lower compartment articles.
- Replace the handwashing articles.
- Close the bag.

Dressing

- Open the bag, take the handwashing articles.
- Open the side pouch, take paper bag, diary, and pen.
- Open the lower compartment, take the kidney tray.
- Remove the old dressing and discard in the kidney tray.
- Do handwashing.
- Open the upper compartment, take the dressing pack consisting of artery forceps, thumb forceps, scissor, cotton balls, gauze piece and needed ointment and solutions.
- Open the dressing pack, take artery forceps, take one cotton and dip it in the normal saline; clean the wound from center to periphery.
- Take another cotton, dip it in the solution and squeeze it in the kidney tray and clean the wound from center to periphery.
- Take the ointment, apply over the wound with the help of cotton.
- Keep the cotton pack, covered with gauze to prevent from sticking to the wound.
- Tie with gauze or put the plaster.
- Clean all the articles if facility available. Boil the water and put the instruments in the water for 10–15 minutes.
- If facility is not available, take one plastic cover and put the used articles inside and sterilize it in health center.
- Do handwashing.
- Replace the upper compartment articles.
- Replace lower compartment articles.
- Replace the handwashing articles.
- Record the procedure.

Oral Medication

- Open the front pouch, take the handwashing articles.
- Open the side pouch, take paper bag.
- Do handwashing.
- Open the upper compartment and take the needed medication.
- Get the water from the client's home and ask the client to open the mouth and swallow the medication with water. Observe that if the client swallowed the medication or not; especially in under fives.
- Discard the waste in the paper bag and burn the paper bag.
- Do handwashing.
- Replace the handwashing articles.
- Close the bag.
- Record the procedure with medicine name, dose, route and action.

Intramuscular Injection (If Standing Order Permitted)

- Open the bag and take the handwashing articles.
- Open the side pouch and take pen, diary and paper bag.
- Do handwashing.
- Open the upper compartment, take the injection pack, which consists of syringe, needle, dry cotton and ampule with cutten. Spirit and needed medication should also be taken.
- Open the pack, take the syringe and needle. Cut the ampule with the help of ampule cutter. If vial, open and take the medicine.
- Select the site, clean with spirit cotton and administer injection intramuscularly.
- Remove the syringe and needle and massage the site.
- Discard the waste in the paper bag and burn the paper bag.
- Clean the articles.

- Do handwashing.
- Replace the articles.
- Record the procedure and observations made.

Cord Care

Prevention of infections is very important, as the newborn infants are not only susceptible but also succumb quickly to infections. The risks are higher in low-birth weight babies, especially preterm.

Purposes

- To prevent infection.
- To promote healing power.
- To clean the cord.

Procedure

1. Take handwashing articles from the bag.
2. Wash hands thoroughly with soap and water.
3. Allow the hands to dry in the air.
4. Get the paper bag ready.
5. Inform the mother.
6. Take out the items needed from sterile compartment.
7. Spread out the central hole towel on the abdomen. Only the cord or umbilicus should be exposed.
8. Keep a small tray containing forceps on the towel.
9. Take the artery forceps and use cotton balls inside the pack.
10. Pour the antiseptic in a small bowl.
11. Clean the cord from center to the periphery.
12. Discard the cotton swab in a paper bag.
13. Repeat the procedure until it is cleaned.
14. Dispose the used swabs by burning or burial.
15. Need not apply any medicine except spirit or Betadine.
16. Do not cover the umbilical cord and leave it open.
17. Wash the items and clean the tray with instruments by using boiling water in the home itself for next use.
18. Wash the hands with soap and water.
19. Replace the articles inside the bag.
20. Give necessary instruction.
21. Plan for next visit.
22. Record the procedure and observations made.

Diabetic Foot Care Procedures

The highest incidents of nontraumatic lower leg amputation involve diabetic patients, according to medical news today. Nerve damage and poor blood flow cause small injuries to quickly escalate. However, amputation is preventable with proper foot care. Keeping a diabetic foot healthy is critical and foot care procedures take only a small amount of time a day.

Inspection

Daily visual foot inspections are recommended. A person with poor eyesight should ask for assistance with foot inspections. Patients should look and feel for any signs of injury. A diabetic must understand that even a small cut or bruise quickly turns into an infected area, if left untreated. Signs of possible foot problems include redness, swelling, foot odor, bruising and loss of hair on toes. Occasionally, a diabetic's foot get fractures, yet the patient remain unaware of the injury because of decreased circulation and sensory loss. A diabetic person may even walk on the fractured foot for several days to weeks without realizing that the foot has become severely injured. Major deformities and further complications may occur. Signs of a foot fracture include redness, increased temperature and change in form or shape. Immediate medical attention is required.

Foot Washing

Wash feet daily with soap and warm water. A diabetic should test water with his hand or wrist prior to placing feet into it. A diabetic's foot may not feel extreme heat and burn/injuries could occur. Rubbing a pumice stone on hard areas of the foot removes the formation of corns and calluses. A person should polish the stone on wet feet. Never attempt cutting calluses off or use chemicals, advises the diabetes foundation. Drying feet thoroughly is important to remove water buildup.

Moisturize

Moisturizing the skin after bathing is critical. A diabetic patient's foot no longer emits oils, which leads to cracking and extreme dryness, explains the diabetes association. The association recommends applying a thin layer of petroleum jelly or other nonfragrance ointment to the foot. A person with diabetes should not apply the lotion between the toes where increased moisture leads to bacterial and fungal growth, which are difficult to heal in a diabetic.

Footwear

Diabetics are discouraged to walk around barefoot due to the increased risk of injury. Soft, seamless socks are encouraged as well as wearing house shoes indoors. A diabetic should always check inside of a shoe for loose pebbles or other items before putting a shoe on. The diabetes association explains that nerves in the foot may have become unable to detect something inside the shoe. Shoes should fit comfortably with enough space around the sides and toes to prevent squeezing from occurring. Special shoes made for diabetic patients are available and often covered by insurance plans.

Health Education

Health education is an essential tool of communication in community health. It has been integrated in all the functions of primary health center.

Purposes

- To motivate people and help them.
- Maintain and adopt good health practices in their daily life.
- To bring out the behavioral changes.
- To inculcate the habits of personal hygiene.

Steps

1. Selection of topic according to the felt needs of the people.
2. Get ready with the articles or necessary audiovisual (AV) aids.
3. Inform the group and motivate them.
4. Speak in an informal way.
5. Select the teaching aids and start with known to unknown.
6. Speak with them in their own language.
7. Select the work area and fix the charts or posters that should be visible to everyone.
8. Use appropriate diagram in the flash card.
9. Use always pointer.
10. Hold the flash cards below the chest level.
11. Explain the story in a narrative form without seeing the cards.
12. Flow of speech should not be disturbed.
13. Make them understand well.
14. Rotate only the body and not to move here and there.
15. Flash cards should be 12–16 in numbers.

16. Follow the principles of AV aids.
17. Encourage participation.
18. Ask questions during health teaching program.

■ THEORIES APPLIED IN COMMUNITY HEALTH NURSING

Introduction

The concept of community is defined as "a group of people who share some important feature of their lives and use some common agencies and institutions." The concept of health is defined as "a balanced state of well-being resulting from harmonious interactions of body, mind and spirit." The term community health is defined by meeting the needs of a community by identifying problems and managing interactions within the community.

Basic Elements

The six basic elements of nursing practice incorporated in community health programs and services are:
1. Promotion of healthful living
2. Prevention of health problem
3. Treatment of disorders
4. Rehabilitation
5. Evaluation
6. Research

Major Roles

The focus of nursing includes not only the individual but also the family and the community; meeting these multiple needs requires multiple roles. The seven major roles of a community health nurse are:
1. Care provider
2. Educator
3. Advocate
4. Manager
5. Collaborator
6. Leader
7. Researcher

Major Settings

Settings for community health nursing can be grouped into six categories:
1. Homes
2. Ambulatory care settings
3. Schools
4. Occupational health settings
5. Residential institutions
6. The community at large
   Community health nursing practice is not limited to a specific area, but can be practiced anywhere.

Theories and Models of Community Health Nursing

The commonly used theories are:
- Nightingale's theory of environment
- Orem's self-care model
- Neuman's healthcare system model
- Roger's model of the science and unitary man

- Pender's health promotion model
- Roy's adaptation model
- Milio's framework for prevention
- Salmon White's construct for public health nursing
- Block and Josten's ethical theory of population-focused nursing
- Canadian model
- Kurt Lewin's theory of social changes

Milio's Framework for Prevention

- Nancy Milio, a nurse and leader in public health policy and public health education, developed a framework for prevention that includes concepts of community-oriented, population-focused care (1976, 1981).
- The basic treatise is that behavioral patterns of populations and individuals who makeup population as a result of habitual selection from limited choices. She challenged the common notion that a main determinant for unhealthful behavioral choice is lack of knowledge. Governmental and institutional policies, set the range of options for personal choice making. It neglected the role of community health nursing, examining the determinants of community health and attempting to influence those determinants through public policy.

Salmon White's Construct for Public Health Nursing

- Mark Salmon White (1982), describes a public health as an organized societal effort to protect, promote and restore the health of people and public health nursing as focused on achieving and maintaining public health.
- He gave three basic priorities practice, i.e., prevention of disease and poor health, protection against disease and external agents and promotion of health. For these three general categories of nursing intervention have also been put forward, these are:
  a. Education directed toward voluntary change in the attitude and behavior of the subjects.
  b. Engineering directed at managing risk-related variables.
  c. Enforcement directed at mandatory regulation to achieve better health.

Scope of prevention spans individual, family, community and global care. Intervention target is in four categories:
1. Human/biological
2. Environmental
3. Medical/technological/organizational
4. Social

Block and Josten's Ethical Theory of Population-focused Nursing

Derryl Block and Lavohn Josten, public health educators, proposed this theory based on intersecting fields of public health and nursing. They have given three essential elements of population-focused nursing that is setup from the first two fields:
1. An obligation to population
2. The primacy of prevention
3. Centrality of relationship-based care
   The first two are from public health and the third element from nursing. Hence, it implies to nursing that relation-based care is very important in population-focused care.

Canadian Model for Community

The community health nurse works with individuals, families, groups, communities, populations, systems and/or society, but at all times the health of the person or community is the focus and motivation from which nursing actions flow. The standards of practice are applied to practice in all settings where people live, work, learn, worship and play.

The philosophical base, foundational values and beliefs that characterize community health nursing—caring the principles of primary healthcare, multiple ways of knowing, individual/community partnerships and empowerment-

are embedded in the standards and are reflected in the development and application of the community health nursing process.

The community health nursing process involves the traditional nursing process components of assessment, planning, intervention and evaluation, but is enhanced by community health nurses in three dimensions:

1. Individual/community participation in each component.
2. Multiple ways of knowing, each of which is necessary to understand the complexity and diversity of nursing in the community. Knowledge and utilization of all these ways of knowing forms evidence-based practice, consistent with these standards.
3. The inherent influence of the broader environment on the individual/community that is the focus of care (e.g., the community will be affected by provincial/territorial policies, its own economic status and by the actions of its individual citizens). The standards of practice are founded on the values and beliefs of community health nurses and utilization of the community health nursing process.

The model illustrates the dynamic nature of community health nursing practice, embracing the present and projecting into the future. The values and beliefs (green or shaded) ground practice in the present, yet guide the evolution of community health nursing practice overtime. The community health nursing process provides the vehicle through which community health nurses work with people and support practice that exemplifies the standards of community health nursing. The standards of practice revolve around both the values and beliefs and the nursing process with the energies of community health nursing always being focused on improving the health of people in the community and facilitating change in systems or society in the support of health. Community health nursing practice does not occur in isolation, but rather within an environmental context, such as policies within their workplace and the legislative framework applicable to their work.

◼ FORMULAE FOR CALCULATION OF IMPORTANT VITAL RATES

$$\text{Neonatal mortality} = \frac{\text{Number of infant death of less than 7 days during the year}}{\text{Number of live birth during the year}} \times 1{,}000$$

$$\text{Neonatal mortality rate (NMR)} = \frac{\text{Number of infant death of less than 28 days during the year}}{\text{Number of live birth during the year}} \times 1{,}000$$

$$\text{Postnatal mortality rate} = \frac{\text{Number of death in particular age group}}{\text{Mid-year population of the same age group}} \times 1{,}000$$

$$\text{Mortality rate (age)} = \frac{\text{Number of death during the year}}{\text{Number of live birth during the year}} \times 1{,}000$$

$$\text{Maternal mortality rate (MMR)} = \frac{\text{Number of maternal death during the year}}{\text{Number of live birth during the year}} \times 1{,}000$$

$$\text{Infant mortality rate (IMR)} = \frac{\text{Number of stillbirth during the year}}{\text{Number of live birth during the year}} \times 1{,}000$$

$$\text{Stillbirth rate (SBR)} = \frac{\text{Number of stillbirth}}{\text{Number of live birth and stillbirth during the year}} \times 1{,}000$$

$$\text{Perinatal mortality rate (PMR)} = \frac{\text{Number of stillbirth and infant deaths}}{\text{Number of live birth and stillbirth during the year}} \times 1{,}000$$

$$\text{Crude birth rate (CBR)} = \frac{\text{Number of live birth during the year}}{\text{Mid-year population}} \times 1{,}000$$

$$\text{Crude death rate (CDR)} = \frac{\text{Number of death during the year}}{\text{Mid-year population}} \times 1{,}000$$

$$\text{Couple protection rate (CPR)} = \frac{\text{Number of ECs protected either by permanent method}}{\text{Total number of eligible couples (ECs)}} \times 1{,}000$$

Or

$$\frac{\text{Temporary method (RU)}}{\text{Total number of ECs}} \times 1{,}000$$

◼ CLASSIFICATION OF PROTEIN-ENERGY MALNUTRITION

Gomez Classification

Protein-energy malnutrition is graded based on the weight, age as percentage of the expected weight as below:

First degree	Weight between 90 and 75% of expected
Second degree	Weight between 75 and 60% of expected
Third degree	Weight below 60% of expected

Wellcome or International Classification

Weight between 60 and 80% of expected:

With edema	Kwashiorkor
Without edema	Undernutrition

Weight below 60% of expected:

With edema	Marasmic kwashiorkor
Without edema	Nutritional marasmus

Classification of Indian Academy of Pediatrics

First degree	Weight between 80 and 70% of expected
Second degree	Weight between 70 and 60% of expected
Third degree	Weight between 60 and 50% of expected
Fourth degree	Weight below 50% of expected

WHO Recommended Nutritive Values for Commonly Used Food Items in India

Sl. No.	Food preparation	Quantity per serving	Weight per serving	Calories (kcal)	Protein (g)	Fat (g)	Carbohy-drates (g)	Calcium (g)	Phospho-rus (g)	Iron (mg)
Cereal and Millet Preparation										
Rice preparation										
1.	Plain rice	2 servings	504	595	11.9	0.9	134.8	0.02	0.2	11.9
2.	Sambar rice	1 serving	485	405	13.5	13.5	76.2	0.08	0.16	13.5
3.	Curd rice	1 serving	253	221	6	7	33.3	0.57	0.10	6
4.	Sweet rice	1 serving	177	432	3.6	12	77.4	0.01	0.05	3.6
5.	Idli	2 pcs	136	130	4.6	0.2	27.6	0.03	0.08	4.6
6.	Plain dosa	2 pcs	100	216	4.1	9.7	28.2	0.03	0.07	4.1
7.	Masala dosa	2 pcs	100	212	4.6	8.4	29.4	0.04	0.08	4.6
8.	Pongal (hot)	1 serving	148	200	5.5	6	30.5	0.03	0.07	5.5
9.	Adai (hot)	1 pc	96	195	6.6	4.4	31.8	0.03	0.09	6.6
Wheat preparation										
1.	Wheat upma	1 serving	128	163	3.8	5.4	24.7	0.01	0.04	0.7
2.	Chapatis	2 pcs	57	196	5	5.5	30.8	0.13	0.02	3
3.	Puris	2 pcs	32	136	2.2	8.4	13	0.06	0.01	1.3
4.	Plain parathas	1 pc	66	104	4.5	19.6	27.3	0.12	0.01	2.7
5.	Rava dosa/Idli	2 pcs	114	212	5	8.5	28.7	0	0.06	0.9
6.	Kesari bath	1 serving	90	284	2	14.6	35.3	0.02	0.04	0.44
7.	Luchi	2 pcs	71	346	4	24	28	0.03	0.01	0.4
Millet preparation										
1.	Ragi balls	1 pc	336	446	6	7.6	86.8	0.3	0.4	6
2.	Ragi roti	2 pcs	185	460	8	9	87	0.3	0.4	6
3.	Maize roti	2 pcs	142	314	9.6	5.5	56.4	0.3	0.1	1.8
4.	Jowar roti	2 pcs	150	252	7.5	1.3	52.5	0.2	0.02	4.5
5.	Ragi puttu	1 plate	146	422	4.4	7.4	84	0.2	0.02	
Pulse preparation										
1.	Bengal gram dal (cooked)	1½ cup	157	284	9	16.4	25.2	0.07	0.13	3.8
2.	Green gram dal (cooked)	1½ cup	142	171	7	7.7	18.4	0.08	0.09	2.7
3.	Red gram dal (cooked)	1½ cup	96	110	6.4	2	16.4	0.05	0.07	2.6
4.	Dal rasam	1½ cup	196	29	1.5	09	38	0.03	0.03	0.09
5.	Radish sambar (sundal)		196	101	4.1	3.6	13.1	0.04	0.07	2.2
6.	Green gram sambar (sundal)	1 plate	142	255	13.5	8.8	30.3	0.05	0.2	2.5
7.	Cowpea sundal	1 plate	142	259	131	9.2	30.9	0.08	0.2	4.8
8.	Amaranth sambar	1½ cup	140	250	5.1	2.7	13	0.05	0.08	8
9.	Bengal gram (sundal)	1 plate	142	272	13.2	11.1	29.7	0.11	0.15	5.5

Contd...

Contd...

Sl. No.	Food preparation	Quantity per serving	Weight per serving	Calories (kcal)	Protein (g)	Fat (g)	Carbohy-drates (g)	Calcium (g)	Phospho-rus (g)	Iron (mg)
Vegetable Preparation										
1.	Amaranth curry	1½ plate	28	47	1.4	2.3	5.1	0.04	0.04	6.64
2.	Amaranth masala	½ plate	42	46	1.2	2.6	44	0.05	0.05	6.8
3.	Brinjal curry	½ plate	45	122	1.4	10.7	4.9	0.02	0.05	0.9
4.	Cabbage and carrot curry	½ plate	56	81	1.5	56	61	0.04	0.12	0.9
Egg, Milk, Meat Preparation										
1.	Meat curry	1 serving	128	220	116	18	2.7	0.1	0.01	2.1
2.	Omelet	1 serving	39	77	5.8	5.7	0.5	0.03	0.1	1
3.	Meat fry	1 serving	142	339	21.8	26	4.5	0.23	0.2	3.3
4.	Fish fry	1 serving	100	220	16.2	16.2	1.4	0.05	0.45	1.2
5.	Rice, mutton pulao	2 servings	341	686	39	39	63.6	0.1	0.22	1.5
6.	Milk (buffalo)	1 cup	200	216	8.4	16	9.2	0.42	0.30	0.8
7.	Milk (cow)	1 cup	200	130	7	9.8	52.7	0.12	0.1	0.4
8.	Buttermilk	1 cup	200	36	1.8	2.8	4.8	0.07	0.07	0.2
9.	Buttermilk (buffalo)	1 cup	200	66	24	5.4	4.8	0.07	0.07	0.2
Preparation Containing Milk										
1.	Coffee	1 cup	200	104	3.8	3.4	14.4	0.1	0.1	1.2
2.	Tea	1 cup	200	72	1.4	1.6	13	0.06	0.04	–
3.	Cocoa	1 cup	200	174	7.5	20.2	20.2	0.2	0.15	0.3
4.	Wheat payasam	1 cup	154	178	3.4	31.5	31.5	0.09	0.08	0.4
5.	Rice payasam	1 cup	266	227	3.7	44.3	44.3	0.14	0.1	4.7
6.	Rice porridge	1 cup	280	263	7.6	44.7	35.9	0.3	0.2	0.7
7.	Bengal gram dal	1 cup	154	178	3.2	35.9	44.7	0.09	0.08	0.4
8.	Soy porridge	1 cup	154	178	7.7	44	44.7	0.07	0.14	0.4
9.	Wheat porridge	1 cup	280	263	7.6	44.7	35.9	0.3	0.22	0.7
10.	Ragi porridge	1 cup	193	317	8.7	52.7	35.9	0.24	0.22	1

Recommended Dietary Allowance (RDA) for Indians

Group	Particulars	Body weight (kg)	Net energy (kcal/ day)	Protein (g/day)	Fat (g/ day)	Calcium g/day	Iron (mg/ day)	Vitamin A (mg/ day)		Thiamine (g/day)	Riboflavin (mg/day)	Nicotinic acid (mg/ day)	Pyridoxine (mg/day)	Ascorbic acid (mg/ day)	Folic acid (mg/ day)	Vitamin B₁₂ (mg/ day)
								Retinol	β-carotene							
Woman	Pregnant	50	+300	+15	30	1,000	38	600	2,400	+0.2	+0.2	+2	2.5	40	400	1
	Lactation 0.6 months	50	+500	+25						+0.3	4 +		2.5	80		
	6–12 months		+400	+18	45	1,000	30	950	3,800	+0.2	+0.2	+3			150	1.5
Infant	0–6 months	5.4	108/kg	2.5/kg						55 mg/ kg	65 mg/kg	170 mg/ kg	0.1			
	6–12 months	8.6	98/kg	1.65/kg		500		350	1,200	50 mg/ kg	60 mg/kg	650 mg/ kg	0.4	25	25	0.2
Children	1–3 years	12.2	1,240	22			12	400		0.6	0.7	8			30	
	4–6 years	19.0	1,690	30	25	400	18	400	1,600	0.9	1.0	11	0.9	40	40	0.2–10
	7–9 years	26.9	1,950	41			26	600	12,400	1.0	1.2	13	1.6		60	

Group	Particulars	Body weight (kg)	Net energy (kcal/ day)	Protein (g/day)	Fat (g/ day)	Calcium g/day	Iron (mg/ day)	Vitamin A (mg/day)		Thiamine (g/day)	Riboflavin (mg/day)	Nicotinic acid (mg/ day)	Pyridoxine (mg/day)	Ascorbic acid (mg/ day)	Folic acid (mg/ day)	Vitamin B₁₂ (mg/ day)
								Retinol	β-carotene							
Boys	10–12 years	35.4	2,190	54			64			1.1	1.3	15				
Girls	10–12 years	31.5	1,970	57	22	600	19	600	2,400	1.0	1.2	13	1.6	40	70	0.2–1.0
Boys	13–15 years	47.8	2,450	70			41			1.2	1.5	16				
Girls	13–15 years	46.7	2,060	65	22	600	28	600	2,400	1.0	1.2	14	2.0	20	100	0.2–1.0
Boys	16–18 years	57.1	2,640	78			50			1.3	1.6	17				
Girls	16–18 years	49.9	2,060	63	22	600	30	600	2,400	1.0	1.2	14	2.0	20	100	0.2–1.0

ESSENTIAL REQUIREMENTS FOR COMMUNITY HEALTH NURSING

Second Year Basic BSc Nursing Programme

Sl. No.	Requirements	Number of requirements	Date of completion of requirements
1.	Orientation report	1	
2.	Community assessment • Rural • Urban	2	
3.	Community survey • Rural • Urban	2	
4.	Household survey	5	
5.	Family folder	5	
6.	Community field visits • Primary health center • Community health center • Sub-center	3	
7.	Nutritional assessment/observation visit • Anganwadi center report • Nutritional assessment of under-five children • Nutritional assessment of antenatal mother • Nutritional assessment of postnatal mother • Nutritional assessment of adult • Nutritional assessment of (others) • Cooking demonstration (1 and 2)	7	
8.	Observation visit • Water purification site • Milk diary • Slaughter house • Sewage disposable site • Rainwater harvesting • Market	6	
9.	Health education/counseling	2	
10.	Preparation of audiovisual aids • Charts • Diorama • Flannel graphs • Flash card • Flip chart • Pamphlet/leaflet • Posters	7	
11.	Family care plan • Rural • Urban	3	
12.	Family care study • Rural • Urban	2	
13.	Biomedical waste management	1	
14.	Records and reports	1	
15.	Notification of epidemic diseases	1	

Contd...

Contd...

Sl. No.	Requirements	Number of requirements	Date of completion of requirements
16.	Communicable and noncommunicable diseases	2	

17.	Bag techniques
	1. Home visit (procedures)
	  – Hand washing technique
	  – Temperature taking
	  – Urine test
		3	

18.	National Health Programme 1. Oral polio programme report 2. Anemia programme report 3. Vitamin A deficiency programme report 4. Diarrhea control programme report 5. Worm infestation control programme report 6. Mental health programme report 7. School health programme report	7	

Signature of Clinical Instructor

Date:

Signature of HOD of Community Health Nursing

Date:

PRACTICAL EXPERIENCE OF COMMUNITY HEALTH NURSING PROGRAMME SCHEDULE

Name of the student   :

Community area   :

Name of the clinical instructor   :

Sl. No.	Date	Activities
1.		
2.		
3.		
4.		
5.		
6.		
7.		
8.		
9.		
10.		
11.		
12.		
13.		
14.		
15.		
16.		
17.		
18.		
19.		
20.		
21.		
22.		
23.		

Contd...

Contd...

Sl. No.	Date	Activities
24.		
25.		
26.		
27.		
28.		
29.		
30.		
31.		
32.		
33.		
34.		
35.		
36.		
37.		
38.		
39.		
40.		

Signature of Clinical Coordinator
Date:

Signature of HOD of Community Health Nursing
Date:

Signature of Principal
Date:

1.1: Orientation Report

Time Schedule and Introduction of Orientation

Members of Group

Number of Groups

Distance from college to PHC

Distance from PHC to Village

Identification of PHC and Route Map of PHC

Total Number of Houses and Type of Houses

Total Population

Area

____

Landmarks

____

Specify the Religious Places

____

Area Map

Signature of the Clinical Instructor
Date:

Signature of HOD of Community Health Nursing
Date:

2.1: Community Assessment (Rural)

Identification Data

1. Name of the area: Rural/urban : _______________________________
2. House number : _______________________________
3. Name of the health center : _______________________________
4. Name of head of the family : _______________________________
5. Family identification : _______________________________
   a. Total number of members in the family : _______________________________
   b. Type of family: Nuclear/ nonnuclear (joint, extended) : _______________________________
   c. Religion : Hindu: __________ Muslim: __________ Christian: __________
      Others: _______________________________
   d. Specify subcaste : _______________________________
   e. Language known : _______________________________
   f. Statement of expenditure of the family:

Items	Amount spent	Expenditure (%)	Items	Amount spent	Expenditure (%)
Food			Clothing		
House rent			Medicine		
Children's education			Recreation (movies, etc.)		
Smoking and/or liquor			Debt		
Savings			Others (specify)		
			Total		

6. Housing condition : _______________________________
   a. Type of house:
      Kutcha: __________ Pucca: __________ Semipucca: __________
   b. Living rooms:
      Number: __________ Adequate: __________ Inadequate: __________
   c. Occupancy: _______________________________
      Tenant: __________ Owner: __________ Monthly rent: __________
   d. Ventilation: _______________________________
      Adequate: __________ Inadequate: __________ No ventilation: __________
   e. Source of lighting: _______________________________
      Electricity: __________ Kerosene: __________ Others (specify): __________
   f. Water supply: _______________________________
      Tube well: __________ Dug well: __________ Lake: __________ Pond: __________
      Municipality water: __________ Others: __________
   g. Kitchen condition: _______________________________
      Separate: __________ Corner of the house: __________ Veranda: __________
   h. Disposal of waste: _______________________________
      Open dumping: __________ Incineration: __________ Manure pits: __________ Others: __________

    i.   Sullage water disposal:

        Open drainage: _________ Closed drain: _________ Soakage pit: _________ Kitchen garden: _________

    ii.   Refuse disposal:

        Indiscriminate throwing: _____________ Garbage: _____________ Compositing: _____________

        Burning: _____________ Municipal collection: _______________ Dumping: _____________

    iii. Excreta disposal:

        Open air defecation: _____________ Separate latrine: _____________ Shared latrine: _____________

        Public toilet: _________________________

7. Family profile:

Sl. No.	Name of the family members	Relation with head	Age in year	Sex	Education	Occupation	Income	Remark on health
1.								
2.								
3.								
4.								
5.								
6.								
7.								

    a.   Total family income per month/year   : _________________________________

8. Transport and communication:

    a.   Transport:

        Own tempo/tractor   : _________________________________

        Use of BMTC/KSRTC/private bus : _________________________________

        Any other   : _________________________________

    b.   Communication:

        Telephone   : _________________________________

        Television   : _________________________________

        Radio   : _________________________________

        Newspaper/magazine   : _________________________________

        Post and telegraph   : _________________________________

9. Dietary pattern:

Food	Food used	Food preparation and storage		
		Traditional	Ideal	Unhygienic
Rice				
Ragi				
Jowar				
Wheat				
Vegetables				
Fish				
Meat				
Egg				
Milk and milk products				
Pulses				
Tubers				
Any others specify				

10. Nutritional status:

Name	Weight (kg)	Height (cm)	Body built				BMI (normal 19–25)		
			Thin	Moderate	Well	Obese	Below normal	Normal	Above normal

   a. Nutritional deficiency:

      Anemic: _______________ Goiter: _______________ Night blindness: _______________

      Scurvy: _______________ Rickets: _______________ Others: _______________

11. Is there any case of fever? If yes, write name, age, treatment with remarks.

   a. With rigors.

   b. With cough.

   c. With rash.

Sl. No.	Name	Age	Discuss	Treatment	Remarks
1.					
2.					
3.					

12. Does anyone have any skin disease (e.g., itching, patch, rash)?

Sl. No.	Name	Age	Discuss	Treatment	Remarks
1.	Itching				
2.	Patch				
3.	Rash				

13. Does anyone have cough more than 1 week?

Sl. No.	Name	Age	Discuss	Treatment	Remarks
1.					
2.					
3.					

14. Does anyone have any other illness?

Sl. No.	Name	Age	Discuss	Treatment	Remarks
1.					
2.					
3.					

15. Is there any woman pregnant? If yes, write the following remarks:

   a. Specify gravida.

   b. Has she been registered?

   c. Is she getting iron and folic acid?

   d. Has she had tetanus toxoid?

Sl. No.	Name	Age	Discuss	Treatment	Remarks
1.					
2.					
3.					

16. Have there been any (within year)—vital statistics?
    a. Births

Sl. No.	Date of birth	Sex	Parents' name	Remarks
1.				
2.				
3.				

    b. Deaths

Sl. No.	Date of death	Sex	Parents' name	Remarks
1.				
2.				
3.				

    c. Marriages

Sl. No.	Date of marriage	Sex	Parents' name	Remarks
1.				
2.				
3.				

17. Are there any children below 5 years who have not received immunization? (Specify name, age, reasons for not immunized in remarks):
    a. BCG vaccination.
    b. DPT vaccination.
    c. Poliomyelitis vaccination.
    d. Measles vaccination.
    e. Vitamin A solution.

Sl. No.	Name	Age	Sex	BCG	DPT			Poliomyelitis	Measles	Vitamin A
					1	2	3			
1.										
2.										
3.										
4.										
5.										

18. Presence of the following:
    a. Mosquitoes: _______________________ House fly: _______________________
    b. Stray dogs: _______________ Cats: _______________ Specify number: _______________
    c. Accident place environment:
       Sharp stones: _______________ Slippery floor: _______________ Stones: _______________
       Open drainage: _______________ Others (specify): _______________

Signature of the Clinical Instructor
Date:

Signature of HOD of Community Health Nursing
Date:

2.2: Community Assessment (Urban)

Identification Data

1. Name of the area: Rural/urban : ____
2. House number : ____
3. Name of the health center : ____
4. Name of head of the family : ____
5. Family identification : ____
   a. Total number of members in the family : ____
   b. Type of family: Nuclear/ non-nuclear (joint, extended) : ____
   c. Religion : Hindu: __________ Muslim: __________ Christian: __________
      Others: ____
   d. Specify subcaste : ____
   e. Language known : ____
   f. Statement of expenditure of the family:

Items	Amount spent	Expenditure (%)	Items	Amount spent	Expenditure (%)
Food			Clothing		
House rent			Medicine		
Children's education			Recreation (movies, etc.)		
Smoking and/or liquor			Debt		
Savings			Others (specify)		
			Total		

6. Housing condition : ____
   a. Type of house:
      Kutcha: __________________ Pucca: __________________ Semipucca: __________________
   b. Living rooms:
      Number: __________________ Adequate: __________________ Inadequate: __________________
   c. Occupancy: ____
      Tenant: __________________ Owner: __________________ Monthly rent: __________________
   d. Ventilation: ____
      Adequate: __________________ Inadequate: __________________ No ventilation: __________________
   e. Source of lighting: ____
      Electricity: __________________ Kerosene: __________________ Others (specify): __________________
   f. Water supply: ____
      Tube well: __________________ Dug well: __________________ Lake: __________________ Pond: __________________
      Municipality water: __________________ Others: __________________
   g. Kitchen condition: ____
      Separate: __________________ Corner of the house: __________________ Veranda: __________________
   h. Disposal of waste: ____
      Open dumping: __________ Incineration: __________ Manure pits: __________ Others: __________
      i. Sullage water disposal:
         Open drainage: __________ Closed drain: __________ Soakage pit: __________ Kitchen garden: __________

ii. Refuse disposal:
   Indiscriminate throwing: _______________ Garbage: _______________ Compositing: _______________
   Burning: _______________ Municipal collection: _______________ Dumping: _______________
iii. Excreta disposal:
   Open air defecation: _______________ Separate latrine: _______________ Sharedlatrine: _______________
   Public toilet: _______________

7. Family profile:

Sl. No.	Name of the family members	Relation with head	Age in year	Sex	Education	Occupation	Income	Remark on health
1.								
2.								
3.								
4.								
5.								
6.								
7.								

a. Total family income per month/year : _______________

8. Transport and communication:
   a. Transport:
      Own tempo/tractor : _______________
      Use of BMTC/KSRTC/private bus : _______________
      Any other : _______________
   b. Communication:
      Telephone : _______________
      Television : _______________
      Radio : _______________
      Newspaper/magazine : _______________
      Post and telegraph : _______________

9. Dietary pattern:

Food	Food used	Food preparation and storage		
		Traditional	Ideal	Unhygienic
Rice				
Ragi				
Jowar				
Wheat				
Vegetables				
Fish				
Meat				
Egg				
Milk and milk products				
Pulses				
Tubers				
Any others specify				

10. Nutritional status:

Name	Weight (kg)	Height (cm)	Body built				BMI (normal 19–25)		
			Thin	Moderate	Well	Obese	Below normal	Normal	Above normal

   a. Nutritional deficiency:
      Anemic: _________________________ Goiter: _________________________ Night blindness: _________________________
      Scurvy: _________________________ Rickets: _________________________ Others: _________________________

11. Is there any case of fever? If yes, write name, age, treatment with remarks.
   a. With rigors.
   b. With cough.
   c. With rash.

Sl. No.	Name	Age	Discuss	Treatment	Remarks
1.					
2.					
3.					

12. Does anyone have any skin disease (e.g., itching, patch, rash)?

Sl. No.	Name	Age	Discuss	Treatment	Remarks
1.	Itching				
2.	Patch				
3.	Rash				

13. Does anyone have cough more than 1 week?

Sl. No.	Name	Age	Discuss	Treatment	Remarks
1.					
2.					
3.					

14. Does anyone have any other illness?

Sl. No.	Name	Age	Discuss	Treatment	Remarks
1.					
2.					
3.					

15. Is there any woman pregnant? If yes, write the following remarks:
   a. Specify gravida.
   b. Has she been registered?
   c. Is she getting iron and folic acid?
   d. Has she had tetanus toxoid?

Sl. No.	Name	Age	Discuss	Treatment	Remarks
1.					
2.					
3.					

16. Have there been any (within year)—vital statistics?
    a. Births

Sl. No.	Date of birth	Sex	Parents' name	Remarks
1.				
2.				
3.				

    b. Deaths

Sl. No.	Date of death	Sex	Parents' name	Remarks
1.				
2.				
3.				

    c. Marriages

Sl. No.	Date of marriage	Sex	Parents' name	Remarks
1.				
2.				
3.				

17. Are there any children below 5 years who have not received immunization? (Specify name, age, reasons for not immunized in remarks):
    a. BCG vaccination.
    b. DPT vaccination.
    c. Poliomyelitis vaccination.
    d. Measles vaccination.
    e. Vitamin A solution.

Sl. No.	Name	Age	Sex	BCG	DPT			Poliomyelitis	Measles	Vitamin A
					1	2	3			
1.										
2.										
3.										
4.										
5.										

18. Presence of the following:
    a. Mosquitoes: ________________________ House fly: ________________________
    b. Stray dogs: ________________ Cats: ________________ Specify number: ________________
    c. Accident place environment:
       Sharp stones: ________________________ Slippery floor: ________________________
       Stones: ________________________ Open drainage: ________________________
       Others (specify): ____

Signature of the Clinical Instructor   **Signature of HOD of Community Health Nursing**

Date: **Date:**

3.1: Community Survey (Rural)

Identification Data

1. Name of the area: Rural/urban : _______________________________________
2. House number : _______________________________________
3. Name of the health center : _______________________________________
4. Name of head of the family : _______________________________________
5. Family identification : _______________________________________
   a. Total number of members in the family : _______________________________________
   b. Type of family: Nuclear/ non-nuclear (joint, extended) : _______________________________________
   c. Religion : Hindu: __________ Muslim: __________ Christian: __________
      Others: __________________________________
   d. Specify subcaste : _______________________________________
   e. Language known : _______________________________________
   f. Statement of expenditure of the family:

Items	Amount spent	Expenditure (%)	Items	Amount spent	Expenditure (%)
Food			Clothing		
House rent			Medicine		
Children's education			Recreation (movies, etc.)		
Smoking and/or liquor			Debt		
Savings			Others (specify)		
			Total		

6. Housing condition : _______________________________________
   a. Type of house:
      Kutcha: __________________ Pucca: __________________ Semipucca: __________________
   b. Living rooms:
      Number: __________________ Adequate: __________________ Inadequate: __________________
   c. Occupancy: _______________________________________
      Tenant: __________________ Owner: __________________ Monthly rent: __________________
   d. Ventilation: _______________________________________
      Adequate: __________________ Inadequate: __________________ No ventilation: __________________
   e. Source of lighting: _______________________________________
      Electricity: __________________ Kerosene: __________________ Others (specify): __________________
   f. Water supply: _______________________________________
      Tube well: __________________ Dug well: __________________ Lake: __________ Pond: __________
      Municipality water: __________________ Others: __________________
   g. Kitchen condition: _______________________________________
      Separate: __________________ Corner of the house: __________________ Veranda: __________________
   h. Disposal of waste: _______________________________________
      Open dumping: __________ Incineration: __________ Manure pits: __________ Others: __________

i. Sullage water disposal:
Open drainage: ___________ Closed drain: ___________ Soakage pit: ___________ Kitchen garden: ___________
ii. Refuse disposal:
Indiscriminate throwing: _______________ Garbage: _______________ Compositing: _______________
Burning: _______________ Municipal collection: _______________ Dumping: _______________
iii. Excreta disposal:
Open air defecation: _______________ Separate latrine: _______________ Shared latrine: _______________
Public toilet: _______________

7. Family profile:

Sl. No.	Name of the family members	Relation with head	Age in year	Sex	Education	Occupation	Income	Remark on health
1.								
2.								
3.								
4.								
5.								
6.								
7.								

a. Total family income per month/year : _______________
8. Transport and communication:
a. Transport:
Own tempo/tractor : _______________
Use of BMTC/KSRTC/private bus : _______________
Any other : _______________
b. Communication:
Telephone : _______________
Television : _______________
Radio : _______________
Newspaper/magazine : _______________
Post and telegraph : _______________
9. Dietary pattern:

Food	Food used	Food preparation and storage		
		Traditional	Ideal	Unhygienic
Rice				
Ragi				
Jowar				
Wheat				
Vegetables				
Fish				
Meat				
Egg				
Milk and milk products				
Pulses				
Tubers				
Any others specify				

10. Nutritional status:

Name	Weight (kg)	Height (cm)	Body built				BMI (normal 19–25)		
			Thin	Moderate	Well	Obese	Below normal	Normal	Above normal

    a. Nutritional deficiency:

        Anemic: ____________________ Goiter: ____________________ Night blindness: ____________________

        Scurvy: ____________________ Rickets: ____________________ Others: ____________________

11. Is there any case of fever? If yes, write name, age, treatment with remarks.

    a. With rigors.

    b. With cough.

    c. With rash.

Sl. No.	Name	Age	Discuss	Treatment	Remarks
1.					
2.					
3.					

12. Does anyone have any skin disease (e.g., itching, patch, rash)?

Sl. No.	Name	Age	Discuss	Treatment	Remarks
1.	Itching				
2.	Patch				
3.	Rash				

13. Does anyone have cough more than 1 week?

Sl. No.	Name	Age	Discuss	Treatment	Remarks
1.					
2.					
3.					

14. Does anyone have any other illness?

Sl. No.	Name	Age	Discuss	Treatment	Remarks
1.					
2.					
3.					

15. Is there any woman pregnant? If yes, write the following remarks:

    a. Specify gravida.

    b. Has she been registered?

    c. Is she getting iron and folic acid?

    d. Has she had tetanus toxoid?

Sl. No.	Name	Age	Discuss	Treatment	Remarks
1.					
2.					
3.					

16. Have there been any (within year)—vital statistics?
    a. Births

Sl. No.	Date of birth	Sex	Parents' name	Remarks
1.				
2.				
3.				

    b. Deaths

Sl. No.	Date of death	Sex	Parents' name	Remarks
1.				
2.				
3.				

    c. Marriages

Sl. No.	Date of marriage	Sex	Parents' name	Remarks
1.				
2.				
3.				

17. Are there any children below 5 years who have not received immunization? (Specify name, age, reasons for not immunized in remarks):
    a. BCG vaccination.
    b. DPT vaccination.
    c. Poliomyelitis vaccination.
    d. Measles vaccination.
    e. Vitamin A solution.

Sl. No.	Name	Age	Sex	BCG	DPT			Poliomyelitis	Measles	Vitamin A
					1	2	3			
1.										
2.										
3.										
4.										
5.										

18. Presence of the following:
    a. Mosquitoes: _________________________ House fly: _________________________
    b. Stray dogs: _______________ Cats: _______________ Specify number: _______________
    c. Accident place environment:
       Sharp stones: _______________ Slippery floor: _______________ Stones: _______________
       Open drainage: _______________ Others (specify): _______________

Signature of the Clinical Instructor
Date:

Signature of HOD of Community Health Nursing
Date:

3.2: Community Survey (Urban)

Identification Data

1. Name of the area: Rural/urban : ____
2. House number : ____
3. Name of the health center : ____
4. Name of head of the family : ____
5. Family identification : ____
   a. Total number of members in
      the family : ____
   b. Type of family: Nuclear/
      non-nuclear (joint, extended) : ____
   c. Religion : Hindu: _________ Muslim: _________ Christian: _________
      Others: ____
   d. Specify subcaste : ____
   e. Language known : ____
   f. Statement of expenditure of the family:

Items	Amount spent	Expenditure (%)	Items	Amount spent	Expenditure (%)
Food			Clothing		
House rent			Medicine		
Children's education			Recreation (movies, etc.)		
Smoking and/or liquor			Debt		
Savings			Others (specify)		
			Total		

6. Housing condition : ____
   a. Type of house:
      Kutcha: _________________ Pucca: _________________ Semipucca: _________________
   b. Living rooms:
      Number: _________________ Adequate: _________________ Inadequate: _________________
   c. Occupancy: ____
      Tenant: _________________ Owner: _________________ Monthly rent: _________________
   d. Ventilation: ____
      Adequate: _________________ Inadequate: _________________ No ventilation: _________________
   e. Source of lighting: ____
      Electricity: _________________ Kerosene: _________________ Others (specify): _________________
   f. Water supply: ____
      Tube well: _________ Dug well: _________ Lake: _________ Pond: _________
      Municipality water: _________________ Others: _________________
   g. Kitchen condition: ____
      Separate: _________________ Corner of the house: _________________ Veranda: _________________
   h. Disposal of waste: ____
      Open dumping: _________ Incineration: _________ Manure pits: _________ Others: _________
      i. Sullage water disposal:
         Open drainage: _________ Closed drain: _________ Soakage pit: _________ Kitchen garden: _________

ii. Refuse disposal:

Indiscriminate throwing: _______________ Garbage: _______________ Compositing: _______________

Burning: _______________ Municipal collection: _______________ Dumping: _______________

iii. Excreta disposal:

Open air defecation: _______________ Separate latrine: _______________ Shared latrine: _______________

Public toilet: _______________

7. Family profile:

Sl. No.	Name of the family members	Relation with head	Age in year	Sex	Education	Occupation	Income	Remark on health
1.								
2.								
3.								
4.								
5.								
6.								
7.								

a. Total family income per month/year : _______________

8. Transport and communication:

a. Transport:

Own tempo/tractor : _______________

Use of BMTC/KSRTC/private bus : _______________

Any other : _______________

b. Communication:

Telephone : _______________

Television : _______________

Radio : _______________

Newspaper/magazine : _______________

Post and telegraph : _______________

9. Dietary pattern:

Food	Food used	Food preparation and storage		
		Traditional	Ideal	Unhygienic
Rice				
Ragi				
Jowar				
Wheat				
Vegetables				
Fish				
Meat				
Egg				
Milk and milk products				
Pulses				
Tubers				
Any others specify				

10. Nutritional status:

Name	Weight (kg)	Height (cm)	Body built				BMI (normal 19–25)		
			Thin	Moderate	Well	Obese	Below normal	Normal	Above normal

    a.   Nutritional deficiency:

        Anemic: _________________ Goiter: _________________ Night blindness: _________________

        Scurvy: _________________ Rickets: _________________ Others: _________________

11. Is there any case of fever? If yes, write name, age, treatment with remarks.

    a.   With rigors.

    b.   With cough.

    c.   With rash.

Sl. No.	Name	Age	Discuss	Treatment	Remarks
1.					
2.					
3.					

12. Does anyone have any skin disease (e.g., itching, patch, rash)?

Sl. No.	Name	Age	Discuss	Treatment	Remarks
1.	Itching				
2.	Patch				
3.	Rash				

13. Does anyone have cough more than 1 week?

Sl. No.	Name	Age	Discuss	Treatment	Remarks
1.					
2.					
3.					

14. Does anyone have any other illness?

Sl. No.	Name	Age	Discuss	Treatment	Remarks
1.					
2.					
3.					

15. Is there any woman pregnant? If yes, write the following remarks:

    a.   Specify gravida.

    b.   Has she been registered?

    c.   Is she getting iron and folic acid?

    d.   Has she had tetanus toxoid?

Sl. No.	Name	Age	Discuss	Treatment	Remarks
1.					
2.					
3.					

16. Have there been any (within year)—vital statistics?
    a. Births

Sl. No.	Date of birth	Sex	Parents' name	Remarks
1.				
2.				
3.				

    b. Deaths

Sl. No.	Date of death	Sex	Parents' name	Remarks
1.				
2.				
3.				

    c. Marriages

Sl. No.	Date of marriage	Sex	Parents' name	Remarks
1.				
2.				
3.				

17. Are there any children below 5 years who have not received immunization? (Specify name, age, reasons for not immunized in remarks):
    a. BCG vaccination.
    b. DPT vaccination.
    c. Poliomyelitis vaccination.
    d. Measles vaccination.
    e. Vitamin A solution.

Sl. No.	Name	Age	Sex	BCG	DPT			Poliomyelitis	Measles	Vitamin A
					1	2	3			
1.										
2.										
3.										
4.										
5.										

18. Presence of the following:
    a. Mosquitoes: _______________________ House fly: _______________________
    b. Stray dogs: _______________ Cats: _______________ Specify number: _______________
    c. Accident place environment:
       Sharp stones: _______________ Slippery floor: _______________
       Stones: _______________ Open drainage: _______________
       Others (specify): _______________

Signature of the Clinical Instructor   **Signature of HOD of Community Health Nursing**

Date: **Date:**

HOUSEHOLD SURVEY – 1

Identification Data

House number : ____

Name of the village : ____

Name of the street : ____

Name of head of the family : ____

Religion : ____

Caste : ____

Type of family : ____

Economic status : ____

Environmental sanitation : ____

Water supply : Adequate/inadequate

Mode of water supply : Tank/well/hand pump

Water source : Protected/unprotected

Refuse disposal : Open dumping/burning/manure pit

Waste water disposal : ___________________________ Stagnation: Yes/No: _____________

If yes, mention type : ____

Excreta disposal : _______________ Latrine: Yes/No: _______________________

If yes, mention type : ____

Family Details

Particulars of the household member

Sl. No.	Name of the family members	Relation with the head of the family	Age	Sex	Marital status	Educational status	Occupational status	Income	Residential status	Health status	Remarks
1.											
2.											
3.											
4.											
5.											
6.											
7.											

Vital Statistics

Birth status

Sl. No.	Name of the child/parent	Date of birth	Sex	Place of birth	Whether registered	Delivery conducted from	Health status of the child	Remarks
1.								
2.								
3.								
4.								
5.								
6.								

Death status

Sl. No.	Name of the deceased person	Age	Sex	Date of death	Place of death	Whether registered	Cause of death	Remarks
1.								
2.								
3.								
4.								

Family welfare—maternal and child health

Sl. No.	Name of the eligible couple	Age at marriage/ whether registered	Number of pregnancy/ pregnancy status	Type of delivery	Infant alive/dead	Age of the infant	Sex of the infant	Birth weight of the infant	Term/ abortion	Any congenital deformities	Remarks
1.											
2.											
3.											
4.											
5.											
6.											

Signature of the Student

Date:

Signature of the Clinical Instructor

Date:

HOUSEHOLD SURVEY – 2

Identification Data

House number : ______________________________________

Name of the village : ______________________________________

Name of the street : ______________________________________

Name of head of the family : ______________________________________

Religion : ______________________________________

Caste : ______________________________________

Type of family : ______________________________________

Economic status : ______________________________________

Environmental sanitation : ______________________________________

Water supply : Adequate/inadequate

Mode of water supply : Tank/well/hand pump

Water source : Protected/unprotected

Refuse disposal : Open dumping/burning/manure pit

Waste water disposal : ______________________ Stagnation: Yes/No: __________

If yes, mention type : ______________________________________

Excreta disposal : ______________ Latrine: Yes/No: __________

If yes, mention type : ______________________________________

Family Details

Particulars of the household member

Sl. No.	Name of the family members	Relation with the head of the family	Age	Sex	Marital status	Educational status	Occupational status	Income	Residential status	Health status	Remarks
1.											
2.											
3.											
4.											
5.											
6.											
7.											

Vital Statistics

Birth status

Sl. No.	Name of the child/parent	Date of birth	Sex	Place of birth	Whether registered	Delivery conducted from	Health status of the child	Remarks
1.								
2.								
3.								
4.								
5.								
6.								

Death status

Sl. No.	Name of the deceased person	Age	Sex	Date of death	Place of death	Whether registered	Cause of death	Remarks
1.								
2.								
3.								
4.								

Family welfare—maternal and child health

Sl. No.	Name of the eligible couple	Age at marriage/ whether registered	Number of pregnancy/ pregnancy status	Type of delivery	Infant alive/dead	Age of the infant	Sex of the infant	Birth weight of the infant	Term/ abortion	Any congenital deformities	Remarks
1.											
2.											
3.											
4.											
5.											
6.											

Signature of the Student

Date:

Signature of the Clinical Instructor

Date:

HOUSEHOLD SURVEY – 3

Identification Data

House number : _______________________________________

Name of the village : _______________________________________

Name of the street : _______________________________________

Name of head of the family : _______________________________________

Religion : _______________________________________

Caste : _______________________________________

Type of family : _______________________________________

Economic status : _______________________________________

Environmental sanitation : _______________________________________

Water supply : Adequate/inadequate

Mode of water supply : Tank/well/hand pump

Water source : Protected/unprotected

Refuse disposal : Open dumping/burning/manure pit

Waste water disposal : _______________________ Stagnation: Yes/No: _______

If yes, mention type : _______________________________________

Excreta disposal : _______________ Latrine: Yes/No: _______________

If yes, mention type : _______________________________________

Family Details

Particulars of the household member

Sl. No.	Name of the family members	Relation with the head of the family	Age	Sex	Marital status	Educational status	Occupational status	Income	Residential status	Health status	Remarks
1.											
2.											
3.											
4.											
5.											
6.											
7.											

Vital Statistics

Birth status

Sl. No.	Name of the child/parent	Date of birth	Sex	Place of birth	Whether registered	Delivery conducted from	Health status of the child	Remarks
1.								
2.								
3.								
4.								
5.								
6.								

Death status

Sl. No.	Name of the deceased person	Age	Sex	Date of death	Place of death	Whether registered	Cause of death	Remarks
1.								
2.								
3.								
4.								

Family welfare—maternal and child health

Sl. No.	Name of the eligible couple	Age at marriage/ whether registered	Number of pregnancy/ pregnancy status	Type of delivery	Infant alive/dead	Age of the infant	Sex of the infant	Birth weight of the infant	Term/ abortion	Any congenital deformities	Remarks
1.											
2.											
3.											
4.											
5.											
6.											

Signature of the Student

Date:

Signature of the Clinical Instructor

Date:

HOUSEHOLD SURVEY – 4

Identification Data

House number : ____

Name of the village : ____

Name of the street : ____

Name of head of the family : ____

Religion : ____

Caste : ____

Type of family : ____

Economic status : ____

Environmental sanitation : ____

Water supply : Adequate/inadequate

Mode of water supply : Tank/well/hand pump

Water source : Protected/unprotected

Refuse disposal : Open dumping/burning/manure pit

Waste water disposal : ______________________ Stagnation: Yes/No: __________

If yes, mention type : ____

Excreta disposal : ______________________ Latrine: Yes/No: __________

If yes, mention type : ____

Family Details

Particulars of the household member

Sl. No.	Name of the family members	Relation with the head of the family	Age	Sex	Marital status	Educational status	Occupational status	Income	Residential status	Health status	Remarks
1.											
2.											
3.											
4.											
5.											
6.											
7.											

Vital Statistics

Birth status

Sl. No.	Name of the child/parent	Date of birth	Sex	Place of birth	Whether registered	Delivery conducted from	Health status of the child	Remarks
1.								
2.								
3.								
4.								
5.								
6.								

Death status

Sl. No.	Name of the deceased person	Age	Sex	Date of death	Place of death	Whether registered	Cause of death	Remarks
1.								
2.								
3.								
4.								

Family welfare—maternal and child health

Sl. No.	Name of the eligible couple	Age at marriage/ whether registered	Number of pregnancy/ pregnancy status	Type of delivery	Infant alive/dead	Age of the infant	Sex of the infant	Birth weight of the infant	Term/ abortion	Any congenital deformities	Remarks
1.											
2.											
3.											
4.											
5.											
6.											

Signature of the Student

Date:

Signature of the Clinical Instructor

Date:

HOUSEHOLD SURVEY – 5

Identification Data

House number : ____

Name of the village : ____

Name of the street : ____

Name of head of the family : ____

Religion : ____

Caste : ____

Type of family : ____

Economic status : ____

Environmental sanitation : ____

Water supply : Adequate/inadequate

Mode of water supply : Tank/well/hand pump

Water source : Protected/unprotected

Refuse disposal : Open dumping/burning/manure pit

Waste water disposal : _________________________ Stagnation: Yes/No: __________

If yes, mention type : ____

Excreta disposal : _____________________ Latrine: Yes/No: __________________

If yes, mention type : ____

Family Details

Particulars of the household member

Sl. No.	Name of the family members	Relation with the head of the family	Age	Sex	Marital status	Educational status	Occupational status	Income	Residential status	Health status	Remarks
1.											
2.											
3.											
4.											
5.											
6.											
7.											

Vital Statistics

Birth status

Sl. No.	Name of the child/parent	Date of birth	Sex	Place of birth	Whether registered	Delivery conducted from	Health status of the child	Remarks
1.								
2.								
3.								
4.								
5.								
6.								

Death status

Sl. No.	Name of the deceased person	Age	Sex	Date of death	Place of death	Whether registered	Cause of death	Remarks
1.								
2.								
3.								
4.								

Family welfare—maternal and child health

Sl. No.	Name of the eligible couple	Age at marriage/ whether registered	Number of pregnancy/ pregnancy status	Type of delivery	Infant alive/dead	Age of the infant	Sex of the infant	Birth weight of the infant	Term/ abortion	Any congenital deformities	Remarks
1.											
2.											
3.											
4.											
5.											
6.											

Signature of the Student

Date:

Signature of the Clinical Instructor

Date:

FAMILY FOLDER – 1

Identification Data

Name of the area: Rural/urban : _______________________________

House number : _______________________________

Name of the health center : _______________________________

Name of head of the family : _______________________________

Family identification : _______________________________

Total number of members in the family : _______________________________

Type of family: Nuclear/
non-nuclear (joint, extended) : _______________________________

Religion : Hindu: __________ Muslim: __________ Christian: __________
Others: _______________________________

Language known : _______________________________

Name of the informer : _______________________________

Age : _______________________________

Sex : _______________________________

Address : _______________________________
: _______________________________
: _______________________________
: _______________________________

Education status : _______________________________

Occupational status : _______________________________

Income of the family : ₹ _______________________________ /month

Family Composition

Sl. No.	Name of the family members	Age	Sex	Relationship with head of the family	Educational status	Occupational status	Health status
1.							
2.							
3.							
4.							
5.							
6.							
7.							
8.							
9.							
10.							
11.							
12.							

Immunization

Immunization chart

Sl. No.	Immunization schedule	Due date	Given date	Weight of the baby/advice
1.	At birth: BCG, OPV			
2.	45 days: DPT, OPV-1st			
3.	75 days: DPT, OPV-2nd			
4.	105 days: DPT, OPV-3rd			
5.	9–10 months: Measles			
6.	18 months: DPT, OPV booster dose			
7.	5 years: DT, OPV			
8.	10 years: TT			
9.	Optional vaccines			
10.				
11.				

Past History of Illness

____
____
____
____
____

Present Complaints

____
____
____
____
____

List Out the Problems and Needs

1. ____
2. ____
3. ____
4. ____
5. ____
6. ____

Problems/needs	Objectives	Nursing interventions	Rationales	Evaluation

Contd...

Contd...

Problems/needs	Objectives	Nursing interventions	Rationales	Evaluation

Contd...

Contd...

Problems/needs	Objectives	Nursing interventions	Rationales	Evaluation

FAMILY FOLDER – 2

Identification Data

Name of the area: Rural/urban : _______________________

House number : _______________________

Name of the health center : _______________________

Name of head of the family : _______________________

Family identification : _______________________

Total number of members in the family : _______________________

Type of family: Nuclear/
non-nuclear (joint, extended) : _______________________

Religion : Hindu: __________ Muslim: __________ Christian: __________
Others: _______________________

Language known : _______________________

Name of the informer : _______________________

Age : _______________________

Sex : _______________________

Address : _______________________
: _______________________
: _______________________
: _______________________

Education status : _______________________

Occupational status : _______________________

Income of the family : ₹ _______________________ /month

Family Composition

Sl. No.	Name of the family members	Age	Sex	Relationship with head of the family	Educational status	Occupational status	Health status
1.							
2.							
3.							
4.							
5.							
6.							
7.							
8.							
9.							
10.							
11.							
12.							

Immunization

Immunization chart

Sl. No.	Immunization schedule	Due date	Given date	Weight of the baby/advice
1.	At birth: BCG, OPV			
2.	45 days: DPT, OPV-1st			
3.	75 days: DPT, OPV-2nd			
4.	105 days: DPT, OPV-3rd			
5.	9–10 months: Measles			
6.	18 months: DPT, OPV booster dose			
7.	5 years: DT, OPV			
8.	10 years: TT			
9.	Optional vaccines			
10.				
11.				

Past History of Illness

____
____
____
____
____

Present Complaints

____
____
____
____
____

List Out the Problems and Needs

1.____
2.____
3.____
4.____
5.____
6.____

Problems/needs	Objectives	Nursing interventions	Rationales	Evaluation

Contd...

Contd...

Problems/needs	Objectives	Nursing interventions	Rationales	Evaluation

Contd...

Contd...

Problems/needs	Objectives	Nursing interventions	Rationales	Evaluation

FAMILY FOLDER – 3

Identification Data

Name of the area: Rural/urban : _______________________________________

House number : _______________________________________

Name of the health center : _______________________________________

Name of head of the family : _______________________________________

Family identification : _______________________________________

Total number of members in the family : _______________________________________

Type of family: Nuclear/
non-nuclear (joint, extended) : _______________________________________

Religion : Hindu: __________ Muslim: __________ Christian: __________

Others: _______________________________________

Language known : _______________________________________

Name of the informer : _______________________________________

Age : _______________________________________

Sex : _______________________________________

Address : _______________________________________

: _______________________________________

: _______________________________________

: _______________________________________

Education status : _______________________________________

Occupational status : _______________________________________

Income of the family : ₹ _______________________________ /month

Family Composition

Sl. No.	Name of the family members	Age	Sex	Relationship with head of the family	Educational status	Occupational status	Health status
1.							
2.							
3.							
4.							
5.							
6.							
7.							
8.							
9.							
10.							
11.							
12.							

Immunization

Immunization chart

Sl. No.	Immunization schedule	Due date	Given date	Weight of the baby/advice
1.	At birth: BCG, OPV			
2.	45 days: DPT, OPV-1st			
3.	75 days: DPT, OPV-2nd			
4.	105 days: DPT, OPV-3rd			
5.	9–10 months: Measles			
6.	18 months: DPT, OPV booster dose			
7.	5 years: DT, OPV			
8.	10 years: TT			
9.	Optional vaccines			
10.				
11.				

Past History of Illness

Present Complaints

List Out the Problems and Needs

1.
2.
3.
4.
5.
6.

Problems/needs	Objectives	Nursing interventions	Rationales	Evaluation

Contd...

Problems/needs	Objectives	Nursing interventions	Rationales	Evaluation

Contd...

Contd...

Problems/needs	Objectives	Nursing interventions	Rationales	Evaluation

FAMILY FOLDER – 4

Identification Data

Name of the area: Rural/urban : _______________________________

House number : _______________________________

Name of the health center : _______________________________

Name of head of the family : _______________________________

Family identification : _______________________________

Total number of members in the family : _______________________________

Type of family: Nuclear/
non-nuclear (joint, extended) : _______________________________

Religion : Hindu: __________ Muslim: __________ Christian: __________

Others: _______________________________

Language known : _______________________________

Name of the informer : _______________________________

Age : _______________________________

Sex : _______________________________

Address : _______________________________

: _______________________________

: _______________________________

: _______________________________

Education status : _______________________________

Occupational status : _______________________________

Income of the family : ₹ _______________________________ /month

Family Composition

Sl. No.	Name of the family members	Age	Sex	Relationship with head of the family	Educational status	Occupational status	Health status
1.							
2.							
3.							
4.							
5.							
6.							
7.							
8.							
9.							
10.							
11.							
12.							

Immunization

Immunization chart

Sl. No.	Immunization schedule	Due date	Given date	Weight of the baby/advice
1.	At birth: BCG, OPV			
2.	45 days: DPT, OPV-1st			
3.	75 days: DPT, OPV-2nd			
4.	105 days: DPT, OPV-3rd			
5.	9–10 months: Measles			
6.	18 months: DPT, OPV booster dose			
7.	5 years: DT, OPV			
8.	10 years: TT			
9.	Optional vaccines			
10.				
11.				

Past History of Illness

Present Complaints

List Out the Problems and Needs

1.

2.

3.

4.

5.

6.

Problems/needs	Objectives	Nursing interventions	Rationales	Evaluation

Contd...

Contd...

Problems/needs	Objectives	Nursing interventions	Rationales	Evaluation

Contd...

Contd...

Problems/needs	Objectives	Nursing interventions	Rationales	Evaluation

FAMILY FOLDER – 5

Identification Data

Name of the area: Rural/urban : _______________________________________

House number : _______________________________________

Name of the health center : _______________________________________

Name of head of the family : _______________________________________

Family identification : _______________________________________

Total number of members in the family : _______________________________________

Type of family: Nuclear/
non-nuclear (joint, extended) : _______________________________________

Religion : Hindu: __________ Muslim: __________ Christian: __________

Others: _______________________________________

Language known : _______________________________________

Name of the informer : _______________________________________

Age : _______________________________________

Sex : _______________________________________

Address : _______________________________________

: _______________________________________

: _______________________________________

: _______________________________________

Education status : _______________________________________

Occupational status : _______________________________________

Income of the family : ₹ ____________________________ /month

Family Composition

Sl. No.	Name of the family members	Age	Sex	Relationship with head of the family	Educational status	Occupational status	Health status
1.							
2.							
3.							
4.							
5.							
6.							
7.							
8.							
9.							
10.							
11.							
12.							

Immunization

Immunization chart

Sl. No.	Immunization schedule	Due date	Given date	Weight of the baby/advice
1.	At birth: BCG, OPV			
2.	45 days: DPT, OPV-1st			
3.	75 days: DPT, OPV-2nd			
4.	105 days: DPT, OPV-3rd			
5.	9–10 months: Measles			
6.	18 months: DPT, OPV booster dose			
7.	5 years: DT, OPV			
8.	10 years: TT			
9.	Optional vaccines			
10.				
11.				

Past History of Illness

Present Complaints

List Out the Problems and Needs

1.
2.
3.
4.
5.
6.

Problems/needs	Objectives	Nursing interventions	Rationales	Evaluation

Contd...

Contd...

Problems/needs	Objectives	Nursing interventions	Rationales	Evaluation

Contd...

Contd...

Problems/needs	Objectives	Nursing interventions	Rationales	Evaluation

6.1: Primary Health Center Report

Introduction of Primary Health Center

Name of the Primary Health Center (PHC)

Aims and Objectives of PHC

Staffing Pattern in PHC

Functions of PHC

____

____

____

____

____

____

Special Days in PHC

____

____

____

____

____

____

Drugs and Equipment Supplies in PHC

____

____

____

____

____

____

Floor Map

Signature of the Clinical Instructor

Date:

Signature of HOD of Community Health Nursing

Date:

Note: During posting, students are observed that they have to write the observation as a PHC report.

6.2: Community Field Visit Center Report

Introduction of Community Health Center

____
____
____
____
____
____
____

Name of the Community Health Center (CHC)

____
____
____
____
____

Aims and Objectives of CHC

____
____
____
____
____

Staffing Pattern in CHC

____
____
____
____
____
____

Functions of CHC

Special Days in CHC

Drugs and Equipment Supplies in CHC

National Health Programme in Community Health Centre

Floor Map

Signature of the Clinical Instructor **Signature of HOD of Community Health Nursing**

Date: **Date:**

Note: During posting, students are observed that they have to write the observation as a CHC report.

6.3: Subcenter Report

Introduction of Subcenter

Name of the Subcenter

Aims and Objectives of Subcenter

Staffing Pattern in Subcenter

Functions of Subcenter

____

____

____

____

____

Special Days in Subcenter

____

____

____

____

____

Drugs and Equipment Supplies in Subcenter

____

____

____

____

____

Floor Map

Signature of the Clinical Instructor   **Signature of HOD of Community Health Nursing**

Date: **Date:**

Note: During posting, students are observed that they have to write the observation as a Sub-Centre report.

7.1: Anganwadi Report

Village name: ____

Anganwadi center name: ____

Anganwadi center no: ____

1. Section: ____

2. Location: ____

3. Infrastructure and equipments : _______________________________

A. Where is the AWC house	1. Own building/permission
	2. Rended building/premises
	3. Anganwadi workers houses
	4. Anganwadi helpers house
	5. Panchayat bhawan
	6. Others (specify)
B. Average distance of Anganwadi from majority of house	
C. The following in place at the AWC and available for ICDS activities	1. Electricity 2. Electric fan 3. Telephone 4. Clean safe drinking water 5. Toilet 6. Indoor activity space 7. Outdoor activity space 8. Kitchen/separate space for cooking 9. Storage facilities for food 10. Storage facilities for equipments

Inventory chart; does the AWC have the following equipments in adequate quantity and satisfactory quality:

Sl. No.	Items	Is it available yes/no	What is the condition good/poor/fair	Remarks
1.	Medicine kit/first aid box			
2.	Baby weighing scale			
3.	Adult weighing scale			
4.	Vessels for cooking			
5.	Indoor play equipments			
6.	Vessels for storing			
7.	Drinking water			

Types of Attendance

	Girls			Boys		
	SC/ST	*Others*	*Total*	*SC/ST*	*Others*	*Total*
Categories						
Infant 0–3 years						
Toddlers 3–6 years						
Mother (pregnant)						
Adolescent girls						

Signature of the Clinical Instructor
Date:

Signature of HOD of Community Health Nursing
Date:

7.2: Nutritional Assessment of Under-five Children

Identification Data

Name of the village/area   : ____

House number   : ____

Name of the family head   : ____

Age   : ____

Sex   : ____

Educational status   : ____

Occupational status   : ____

Address   : ____

____

Common cooking method   : Steaming/boiling/deep or shallow frying

Preparation of food   : Hygienic/unhygienic

Commonly consuming food items   : ____

: ____

Particulars of Parents

Sl. No.	Name of the parents	Age	Sex	Education	Occupation	Remarks
1.						
2.						

Number of Living Children

Sl. No.	Name of the children	Order of live birth	Date of birth	Age	Sex	Education
1.						
2.						
3.						

Anthropometric Measurements

Weight (kg)   : ____

Height or length (cm)   : ____

Head circumference (cm)   : ____

Chest circumference (cm)   : ____

Midarm circumference (cm)   : ____

Degree of Malnutrition

Body Mass Index

Growth Chart

Twenty Four-hour Dietary Recall Survey

Name of the area   : ____

Taluk   : ____

District   : ____

Religion   : ____

Total number of family members : ____

Family income   : ____

Family Characteristics

Sl. No.	Name	Age	Occupation			Vegetarian	Nonvegetarian
			Sedentary	Moderate	Hard		
1.							
2.							
3.							
4.							
5.							
6.							

Purchase of Raw Material and Their Expenditure Per Day

Items	How often purchasing?			Monthly	Seasonally	Quantity	Expenditure per day
	Daily	Biweekly	Weekly				
Cereals							
Pulses							
Milk							
Fruits							
Vegetables							
Jaggery							
Sugar							
Ghee							
Oil							
Eggs							
Meat							
Fish							

Shopping facilities   : Market/village shop/sunday market/any other forms

Preservation of raw foods   : Store room/kitchen/no store/living room

Preservation of cooked foods : Refrigerator/cupboard/kitchen

Fuel used for cooking   : Cooking gas/electrical stove/firewood/kerosene stove

Do You Have

Vegetable garden   : ____

Fruit tree   : ____

Household Animals

Cow   : ____

Buffalo   : ____

Hen   : ____

Goat   : ____

Pig   : ____

Nutrition Cycle of the Family

Items/days	Items in grams							Average daily intake	Category
	1	2	3	4	5	6	7		
Wheat									Cereals
Rice									
Jowar									
Bajara									
Other									
Toor dal									Pulses
Arhar									
Urad									
Moong									
Green gram									
Groundnuts									
Others									
Milk									Milk products
Curd									
Buttermilk									
Others									
Oil									Fats
Ghee									
Dalda									
Leafy vegetables									Vegetables
Root/tubers									
Others									
Tea									Beverages
Coffee									
Others									
Sugar									Sugar
Jaggery									
Meat									Nonvegetarian
Fish									
Egg									

Contd...

Contd...

Items/days	Items in grams							Average daily intake	Category
	1	2	3	4	5	6	7		
Banana									Fruits
Orange									
Papaya									
Pineapple									
Grapes									
Apple									
Guava									
Others									

Inference

____

____

____

____

____

____

____

____

____

____

____

____

____

____

____

____

____

____

____

____

____

____

WHO Recommended Nutritive Values for Commonly Used Food Items in India

Sl. No.	Food preparation	Quantity per serving	Weight per serving	Calories (kcal)	Protein (g)	Fat (g)	Carbohydrates (g)	Calcium (g)	Phospho-rus (g)	Iron (mg)
Cereal and Millet Preparation										
Rice preparation										
1.	Plain rice	2 servings	504	595	11.9	0.9	134.8	0.02	0.2	11.9
2.	Sambar rice	1 serving	485	405	13.5	13.5	76.2	0.08	0.16	13.5
3.	Curd rice	1 serving	253	221	6	7	33.3	0.57	0.10	6
4.	Sweet rice	1 serving	177	432	3.6	12	77.4	0.01	0.05	3.6
5.	Idli	2 pcs	136	130	4.6	0.2	27.6	0.03	0.08	4.6
6.	Plain dosa	2 pcs	100	216	4.1	9.7	28.2	0.03	0.07	4.1
7.	Masala dosa	2 pcs	100	212	4.6	8.4	29.4	0.04	0.08	4.6
8.	Pongal (hot)	1 serving	148	200	5.5	6	30.5	0.03	0.07	5.5
9.	Adai (hot)	1 pc	96	195	6.6	4.4	31.8	0.03	0.09	6.6
Wheat preparation										
1.	Wheat upma	1 serving	128	163	3.8	5.4	24.7	0.01	0.04	0.7
2.	Chapatis	2 pcs	57	196	5	5.5	30.8	0.13	0.02	3
3.	Puris	2 pcs	32	136	2.2	8.4	13	0.06	0.01	1.3
4.	Plain parathas	1 pc	66	104	4.5	19.6	27.3	0.12	0.01	2.7
5.	Rava dosa/Idli	2 pcs	114	212	5	8.5	28.7	0	0.06	0.9
6.	Kesari bath	1 serving	90	284	2	14.6	35.3	0.02	0.04	0.44
7.	Luchi	2 pcs	71	346	4	24	28	0.03	0.01	0.4
Millet preparation										
1.	Ragi balls	1 pc	336	446	6	7.6	86.8	0.3	0.4	6
2.	Ragi roti	2 pcs	185	460	8	9	87	0.3	0.4	6
3.	Maize roti	2 pcs	142	314	9.6	5.5	56.4	0.3	0.1	1.8
4.	Jowar roti	2 pcs	150	252	7.5	1.3	52.5	0.2	0.02	4.5
5.	Ragi puttu	1 plate	146	422	4.4	7.4	84	0.2	0.02	-
Pulse preparation										
1.	Bengal gram dal (cooked)	1½ cup	157	284	9	16.4	25.2	0.07	0.13	3.8
2.	Green gram dal (cooked)	1½ cup	142	171	7	7.7	18.4	0.08	0.09	2.7
3.	Red gram dal (cooked)	1½ cup	96	110	6.4	2	16.4	0.05	0.07	2.6
4.	Dal rasam	1½ cup	196	29	1.5	0.9	38	0.03	0.03	0.09
5.	Radish sambar (sundal)		196	101	4.1	3.6	13.1	0.04	0.07	2.2
6.	Green gram sambar (sundal)	1 plate	142	255	13.5	8.8	30.3	0.05	0.2	2.5
7.	Cowpea sundal	1 plate	142	259	13.1	9.2	30.9	0.08	0.2	4.8
8.	Amaranth sambar	1½ cup	140	250	5.1	2.7	13	0.05	0.08	8
9.	Bengal gram (sundal)	1 plate	142	272	13.2	11.1	29.7	0.11	0.15	5.5
Vegetable Preparation										
1.	Amaranth curry	1½ plate	28	47	1.4	2.3	5.1	0.04	0.04	6.64
2.	Amaranth masala	½ plate	42	46	1.2	2.6	44	0.05	0.05	6.8

Contd...

Contd...

Sl. No.	Food preparation	Quantity per serving	Weight per serving	Calories (kcal)	Protein (g)	Fat (g)	Carbohydrates (g)	Calcium (g)	Phosphorus (g)	Iron (mg)
3.	Brinjal curry	½ plate	45	122	1.4	10.7	4.9	0.02	0.05	0.9
4.	Cabbage and carrot curry	½ plate	56	81	1.5	56	61	0.04	0.12	0.9
Egg, Milk, and Meat Preparation										
1.	Meat curry	1 serving	128	220	116	18	2.7	0.1	0.01	2.1
2.	Omelet	1 serving	39	77	5.8	5.7	0.5	0.03	0.1	1
3.	Meat fry	1 serving	142	339	21.8	26	4.5	0.23	0.2	3.3
4.	Fish fry	1 serving	100	220	16.2	16.2	1.4	0.05	0.45	1.2
5.	Rice, mutton pulav	2 servings	341	686	39	39	63.6	0.1	0.22	1.5
6.	Milk (buffalo)	1 cup	200	216	8.4	16	9.2	0.42	0.30	0.8
7.	Milk (cow)	1 cup	200	130	7	9.8	52.7	0.12	0.1	0.4
8.	Buttermilk	1 cup	200	36	1.8	2.8	4.8	0.07	0.07	0.2
9.	Buttermilk (buffalo)	1 cup	200	66	24	5.4	4.8	0.07	0.07	0.2
Preparation Containing Milk										
1.	Coffee	1 cup	200	104	3.8	3.4	14.4	0.1	0.1	1.2
2.	Tea	1 cup	200	72	1.4	1.6	13	0.06	0.04	-
3.	Cocoa	1 cup	200	174	7.5	20.2	20.2	0.2	0.15	0.3
4.	Wheat payasam	1 cup	154	178	3.4	31.5	31.5	0.09	0.08	0.4
5.	Rice payasam	1 cup	266	227	3.7	44.3	44.3	0.14	0.1	4.7
6.	Rice porridge	1 cup	280	263	7.6	44.7	35.9	0.3	0.2	0.7
7.	Bengal gram dal	1 cup	154	178	3.2	35.9	44.7	0.09	0.08	0.4
8.	Soy porridge	1 cup	154	178	7.7	44	44.7	0.07	0.14	0.4
9.	Wheat porridge	1 cup	280	263	7.6	44.7	35.9	0.3	0.22	0.7
10.	Ragi porridge	1 cup	193	317	8.7	52.7	35.9	0.24	0.22	1

7.3: Nutritional Assessment of Antenatal Mother

Identification Data

Name of the village/area : _______________________________

House number : _______________________________

Name of the family head : _______________________________

Age : _______________________________

Sex : _______________________________

Educational status : _______________________________

Occupational status : _______________________________

Address : _______________________________

Common cooking method : Steaming/boiling/deep or shallow frying

Preparation of food : Hygienic/unhygienic

Commonly consuming food items : _______________________________

: _______________________________

Particulars of Parents

Sl. No.	Name of the parents	Age	Sex	Education	Occupation	Remarks
1.						
2.						

Number of Living Children

Sl. No.	Name of the children	Order of live birth	Date of birth	Age	Sex	Education
1.						
2.						
3.						

Anthropometric Measurements

Weight (kg) : _______________________________

Height or length (cm) : _______________________________

Head circumference (cm) : _______________________________

Chest circumference (cm) : _______________________________

Midarm circumference (cm) : _______________________________

Degree of Malnutrition

Body Mass Index

Growth Chart

Twenty Four-hour Dietary Recall Survey

Name of the area   : _______________________________

Taluk   : _______________________________

District   : _______________________________

Religion   : _______________________________

 Total number of family members   : _______________________________

Family income   : _______________________________

Family Characteristics

Sl. No.	Name	Age	Occupation			Vegetarian	Nonvegetarian
			Sedentary	Moderate	Hard		
1.							
2.							
3.							
4.							
5.							
6.							

Purchase of Raw Material and Their Expenditure Per Day

Items	How often purchasing?			Monthly	Seasonally	Quantity	Expenditure per day
	Daily	Biweekly	Weekly				
Cereals							
Pulses							
Milk							
Fruits							
Vegetables							
Jaggery							
Sugar							
Ghee							
Oil							
Eggs							
Meat							
Fish							

Shopping facilities   : Market/village shop/sunday market/any other forms
Preservation of raw foods   : Store room/kitchen/no store/living room
Preservation of cooked foods   : Refrigerator/cupboard/kitchen
Fuel used for cooking   : Cooking gas/electrical stove/firewood/kerosene stove

Do You Have

Vegetable garden   : _______________________________

Fruit tree   : _______________________________

Household Animals

Cow   :____

Buffalo   :____

Hen   :____

Goat   :____

Pig   :____

Nutrition Cycle of the Family

Items/days	Items in grams							Average daily intake	Category
	1	2	3	4	5	6	7		
Wheat									Cereals
Rice									
Jowar									
Bajara									
Other									
Toor dal									Pulses
Arhar									
Urad									
Moong									
Green gram									
Groundnuts									
Others									
Milk									Milk products
Curd									
Buttermilk									
Others									
Oil									Fats
Ghee									
Dalda									
Leafy vegetables									Vegetables
Root/tubers									
Others									
Tea									Beverages
Coffee									
Others									
Sugar									Sugar
Jaggery									
Meat									Nonvegetarian
Fish									
Egg									

Contd...

Contd...

Items/days	Items in grams							Average daily intake	Category
	1	**2**	**3**	**4**	**5**	**6**	**7**		
Banana									Fruits
Orange									
Papaya									
Pineapple									
Grapes									
Apple									
Guava									
Others									

Inference

____

____

____

____

____

____

____

____

____

____

____

____

____

____

____

____

____

____

____

____

____

____

WHO Recommended Nutritive Values for Commonly Used Food Items in India

Sl. No.	Food preparation	Quantity per serving	Weight per serving	Calories (kcal)	Protein (g)	Fat (g)	Carbohydrates (g)	Calcium (g)	Phospho-rus (g)	Iron (mg)
Cereal and Millet Preparation										
Rice preparation										
1.	Plain rice	2 servings	504	595	11.9	0.9	134.8	0.02	0.2	11.9
2.	Sambar rice	1 serving	485	405	13.5	13.5	76.2	0.08	0.16	13.5
3.	Curd rice	1 serving	253	221	6	7	33.3	0.57	0.10	6
4.	Sweet rice	1 serving	177	432	3.6	12	77.4	0.01	0.05	3.6
5.	Idli	2 pcs	136	130	4.6	0.2	27.6	0.03	0.08	4.6
6.	Plain dosa	2 pcs	100	216	4.1	9.7	28.2	0.03	0.07	4.1
7.	Masala dosa	2 pcs	100	212	4.6	8.4	29.4	0.04	0.08	4.6
8.	Pongal (hot)	1 serving	148	200	5.5	6	30.5	0.03	0.07	5.5
9.	Adai (hot)	1 pc	96	195	6.6	4.4	31.8	0.03	0.09	6.6
Wheat preparation										
1.	Wheat upma	1 serving	128	163	3.8	5.4	24.7	0.01	0.04	0.7
2.	Chapatis	2 pcs	57	196	5	5.5	30.8	0.13	0.02	3
3.	Puris	2 pcs	32	136	2.2	8.4	13	0.06	0.01	1.3
4.	Plain parathas	1 pc	66	104	4.5	19.6	27.3	0.12	0.01	2.7
5.	Rava dosa/Idli	2 pcs	114	212	5	8.5	28.7	0	0.06	0.9
6.	Kesari bath	1 serving	90	284	2	14.6	35.3	0.02	0.04	0.44
7.	Luchi	2 pcs	71	346	4	24	28	0.03	0.01	0.4
Millet preparation										
1.	Ragi balls	1 pc	336	446	6	7.6	86.8	0.3	0.4	6
2.	Ragi roti	2 pcs	185	460	8	9	87	0.3	0.4	6
3.	Maize roti	2 pcs	142	314	9.6	5.5	56.4	0.3	0.1	1.8
4.	Jowar roti	2 pcs	150	252	7.5	1.3	52.5	0.2	0.02	4.5
5.	Ragi puttu	1 plate	146	422	4.4	7.4	84	0.2	0.02	-
Pulse preparation										
1.	Bengal gram dal (cooked)	1½ cup	157	284	9	16.4	25.2	0.07	0.13	3.8
2.	Green gram dal (cooked)	1½ cup	142	171	7	7.7	18.4	0.08	0.09	2.7
3.	Red gram dal (cooked)	1½ cup	96	110	6.4	2	16.4	0.05	0.07	2.6
4.	Dal rasam	1½ cup	196	29	1.5	0.9	38	0.03	0.03	0.09
5.	Radish sambar (sundal)		196	101	4.1	3.6	13.1	0.04	0.07	2.2
6.	Green gram sambar (sundal)	1 plate	142	255	13.5	8.8	30.3	0.05	0.2	2.5
7.	Cowpea sundal	1 plate	142	259	13.1	9.2	30.9	0.08	0.2	4.8
8.	Amaranth sambar	1½ cup	140	250	5.1	2.7	13	0.05	0.08	8
9.	Bengal gram (sundal)	1 plate	142	272	13.2	11.1	29.7	0.11	0.15	5.5
Vegetable Preparation										
1.	Amaranth curry	1½ plate	28	47	1.4	2.3	5.1	0.04	0.04	6.64
2.	Amaranth masala	½ plate	42	46	1.2	2.6	44	0.05	0.05	6.8

Contd...

Contd...

Sl. No.	Food preparation	Quantity per serving	Weight per serving	Calories (kcal)	Protein (g)	Fat (g)	Carbohydrates (g)	Calcium (g)	Phosphorus (g)	Iron (mg)
3.	Brinjal curry	½ plate	45	122	1.4	10.7	4.9	0.02	0.05	0.9
4.	Cabbage and carrot curry	½ plate	56	81	1.5	56	61	0.04	0.12	0.9
Egg, Milk, and Meat Preparation										
1.	Meat curry	1 serving	128	220	116	18	2.7	0.1	0.01	2.1
2.	Omelet	1 serving	39	77	5.8	5.7	0.5	0.03	0.1	1
3.	Meat fry	1 serving	142	339	21.8	26	4.5	0.23	0.2	3.3
4.	Fish fry	1 serving	100	220	16.2	16.2	1.4	0.05	0.45	1.2
5.	Rice, mutton pulav	2 servings	341	686	39	39	63.6	0.1	0.22	1.5
6.	Milk (buffalo)	1 cup	200	216	8.4	16	9.2	0.42	0.30	0.8
7.	Milk (cow)	1 cup	200	130	7	9.8	52.7	0.12	0.1	0.4
8.	Buttermilk	1 cup	200	36	1.8	2.8	4.8	0.07	0.07	0.2
9.	Buttermilk (buffalo)	1 cup	200	66	24	5.4	4.8	0.07	0.07	0.2
Preparation Containing Milk										
1.	Coffee	1 cup	200	104	3.8	3.4	14.4	0.1	0.1	1.2
2.	Tea	1 cup	200	72	1.4	1.6	13	0.06	0.04	-
3.	Cocoa	1 cup	200	174	7.5	20.2	20.2	0.2	0.15	0.3
4.	Wheat payasam	1 cup	154	178	3.4	31.5	31.5	0.09	0.08	0.4
5.	Rice payasam	1 cup	266	227	3.7	44.3	44.3	0.14	0.1	4.7
6.	Rice porridge	1 cup	280	263	7.6	44.7	35.9	0.3	0.2	0.7
7.	Bengal gram dal	1 cup	154	178	3.2	35.9	44.7	0.09	0.08	0.4
8.	Soy porridge	1 cup	154	178	7.7	44	44.7	0.07	0.14	0.4
9.	Wheat porridge	1 cup	280	263	7.6	44.7	35.9	0.3	0.22	0.7
10.	Ragi porridge	1 cup	193	317	8.7	52.7	35.9	0.24	0.22	1

7.4: Nutritional Assessment of Postnatal Mother

Identification Data

Name of the village/area   : ______________________________

House number   : ______________________________

Name of the family head   : ______________________________

Age   : ______________________________

Sex   : ______________________________

Educational status   : ______________________________

Occupational status   : ______________________________

Address   : ______________________________

                                 ____

Common cooking method   : Steaming/boiling/deep or shallow frying

Preparation of food   : Hygienic/unhygienic

Commonly consuming food items : ______________________________

                                 : ______________________________

Particulars of Parents

Sl. No.	Name of the parents	Age	Sex	Education	Occupation	Remarks
1.						
2.						

Number of Living Children

Sl. No.	Name of the children	Order of live birth	Date of birth	Age	Sex	Education
1.						
2.						
3.						

Anthropometric Measurements

Weight (kg)   : ______________________________

Height or length (cm)   : ______________________________

Head circumference (cm)   : ______________________________

Chest circumference (cm)   : ______________________________

Midarm circumference (cm)   : ______________________________

Degree of Malnutrition

____

____

____

____

____

____

____

____

____

Body Mass Index

____

____

____

____

____

____

____

____

____

Growth Chart

Twenty Four-hour Dietary Recall Survey

Name of the area   : ___________________________________

Taluk   : ___________________________________

District   : ___________________________________

Religion   : ___________________________________

Total number of family members : ___________________________________

Family income   : ___________________________________

Family Characteristics

Sl. No.	Name	Age	Occupation			Vegetarian	Nonvegetarian
			Sedentary	Moderate	Hard		
1.							
2.							
3.							
4.							
5.							
6.							

Purchase of Raw Material and Their Expenditure Per Day

Items	How often purchasing?			Monthly	Seasonally	Quantity	Expenditure per day
	Daily	Biweekly	Weekly				
Cereals							
Pulses							
Milk							
Fruits							
Vegetables							
Jaggery							
Sugar							
Ghee							
Oil							
Eggs							
Meat							
Fish							

Shopping facilities   : Market/village shop/sunday market/any other forms
Preservation of raw foods   : Store room/kitchen/no store/living room
Preservation of cooked foods : Refrigerator/cupboard/kitchen
Fuel used for cooking   : Cooking gas/electrical stove/firewood/kerosene stove

Do You Have

Vegetable garden   : ___________________________________
Fruit tree   : ___________________________________

Household Animals

Cow : ____

Buffalo : ____

Hen : ____

Goat : ____

Pig : ____

Nutrition Cycle of the Family

Items/days	Items in grams							Average daily intake	Category
	1	2	3	4	5	6	7		
Wheat									Cereals
Rice									
Jowar									
Bajara									
Other									
Toor dal									Pulses
Arhar									
Urad									
Moong									
Green gram									
Groundnuts									
Others									
Milk									Milk products
Curd									
Buttermilk									
Others									
Oil									Fats
Ghee									
Dalda									
Leafy vegetables									Vegetables
Root/tubers									
Others									
Tea									Beverages
Coffee									
Others									
Sugar									Sugar
Jaggery									
Meat									Nonvegetarian
Fish									
Egg									

Contd...

Contd...

Items/days	Items in grams							Average daily intake	Category
	1	2	3	4	5	6	7		
Banana									Fruits
Orange									
Papaya									
Pineapple									
Grapes									
Apple									
Guava									
Others									

Inference

____
____
____
____
____
____
____
____
____
____
____
____
____
____
____
____
____
____
____
____
____
____
____

WHO Recommended Nutritive Values for Commonly Used Food Items in India

Sl. No.	Food preparation	Quantity per serving	Weight per serving	Calories (kcal)	Protein (g)	Fat (g)	Carbohydrates (g)	Calcium (g)	Phosphorus (g)	Iron (mg)
Cereal and Millet Preparation										
Rice preparation										
1.	Plain rice	2 servings	504	595	11.9	0.9	134.8	0.02	0.2	11.9
2.	Sambar rice	1 serving	485	405	13.5	13.5	76.2	0.08	0.16	13.5
3.	Curd rice	1 serving	253	221	6	7	33.3	0.57	0.10	6
4.	Sweet rice	1 serving	177	432	3.6	12	77.4	0.01	0.05	3.6
5.	Idli	2 pcs	136	130	4.6	0.2	27.6	0.03	0.08	4.6
6.	Plain dosa	2 pcs	100	216	4.1	9.7	28.2	0.03	0.07	4.1
7.	Masala dosa	2 pcs	100	212	4.6	8.4	29.4	0.04	0.08	4.6
8.	Pongal (hot)	1 serving	148	200	5.5	6	30.5	0.03	0.07	5.5
9.	Adai (hot)	1 pc	96	195	6.6	4.4	31.8	0.03	0.09	6.6
Wheat preparation										
1.	Wheat upma	1 serving	128	163	3.8	5.4	24.7	0.01	0.04	0.7
2.	Chapatis	2 pcs	57	196	5	5.5	30.8	0.13	0.02	3
3.	Puris	2 pcs	32	136	2.2	8.4	13	0.06	0.01	1.3
4.	Plain parathas	1 pc	66	104	4.5	19.6	27.3	0.12	0.01	2.7
5.	Rava dosa/Idli	2 pcs	114	212	5	8.5	28.7	0	0.06	0.9
6.	Kesari bath	1 serving	90	284	2	14.6	35.3	0.02	0.04	0.44
7.	Luchi	2 pcs	71	346	4	24	28	0.03	0.01	0.4
Millet preparation										
1.	Ragi balls	1 pc	336	446	6	7.6	86.8	0.3	0.4	6
2.	Ragi roti	2 pcs	185	460	8	9	87	0.3	0.4	6
3.	Maize roti	2 pcs	142	314	9.6	5.5	56.4	0.3	0.1	1.8
4.	Jowar roti	2 pcs	150	252	7.5	1.3	52.5	0.2	0.02	4.5
5.	Ragi puttu	1 plate	146	422	4.4	7.4	84	0.2	0.02	–
Pulse preparation										
1.	Bengal gram dal (cooked)	1½ cup	157	284	9	16.4	25.2	0.07	0.13	3.8
2.	Green gram dal (cooked)	1½ cup	142	171	7	7.7	18.4	0.08	0.09	2.7
3.	Red gram dal (cooked)	1½ cup	96	110	6.4	2	16.4	0.05	0.07	2.6
4.	Dal rasam	1½ cup	196	29	1.5	0.9	38	0.03	0.03	0.09
5.	Radish sambar (sundal)		196	101	4.1	3.6	13.1	0.04	0.07	2.2
6.	Green gram sambar (sundal)	1 plate	142	255	13.5	8.8	30.3	0.05	0.2	2.5
7.	Cowpea sundal	1 plate	142	259	13.1	9.2	30.9	0.08	0.2	4.8
8.	Amaranth sambar	1½ cup	140	250	5.1	2.7	13	0.05	0.08	8
9.	Bengal gram (sundal)	1 plate	142	272	13.2	11.1	29.7	0.11	0.15	5.5
Vegetable Preparation										
1.	Amaranth curry	1½ plate	28	47	1.4	2.3	5.1	0.04	0.04	6.64
2.	Amaranth masala	½ plate	42	46	1.2	2.6	44	0.05	0.05	6.8

Contd...

Contd...

Sl. No.	Food preparation	Quantity per serving	Weight per serving	Calories (kcal)	Protein (g)	Fat (g)	Carbohydrates (g)	Calcium (g)	Phospho-rus (g)	Iron (mg)
3.	Brinjal curry	½ plate	45	122	1.4	10.7	4.9	0.02	0.05	0.9
4.	Cabbage and carrot curry	½ plate	56	81	1.5	56	61	0.04	0.12	0.9
Egg, Milk, and Meat Preparation										
1.	Meat curry	1 serving	128	220	116	18	2.7	0.1	0.01	2.1
2.	Omelet	1 serving	39	77	5.8	5.7	0.5	0.03	0.1	1
3.	Meat fry	1 serving	142	339	21.8	26	4.5	0.23	0.2	3.3
4.	Fish fry	1 serving	100	220	16.2	16.2	1.4	0.05	0.45	1.2
5.	Rice, mutton pulav	2 servings	341	686	39	39	63.6	0.1	0.22	1.5
6.	Milk (buffalo)	1 cup	200	216	8.4	16	9.2	0.42	0.30	0.8
7.	Milk (cow)	1 cup	200	130	7	9.8	52.7	0.12	0.1	0.4
8.	Buttermilk	1 cup	200	36	1.8	2.8	4.8	0.07	0.07	0.2
9.	Buttermilk (buffalo)	1 cup	200	66	24	5.4	4.8	0.07	0.07	0.2
Preparation Containing Milk										
1.	Coffee	1 cup	200	104	3.8	3.4	14.4	0.1	0.1	1.2
2.	Tea	1 cup	200	72	1.4	1.6	13	0.06	0.04	-
3.	Cocoa	1 cup	200	174	7.5	20.2	20.2	0.2	0.15	0.3
4.	Wheat payasam	1 cup	154	178	3.4	31.5	31.5	0.09	0.08	0.4
5.	Rice payasam	1 cup	266	227	3.7	44.3	44.3	0.14	0.1	4.7
6.	Rice porridge	1 cup	280	263	7.6	44.7	35.9	0.3	0.2	0.7
7.	Bengal gram dal	1 cup	154	178	3.2	35.9	44.7	0.09	0.08	0.4
8.	Soy porridge	1 cup	154	178	7.7	44	44.7	0.07	0.14	0.4
9.	Wheat porridge	1 cup	280	263	7.6	44.7	35.9	0.3	0.22	0.7
10.	Ragi porridge	1 cup	193	317	8.7	52.7	35.9	0.24	0.22	1

7.5: Nutritional Assessment of Adult

Identification Data

Name of the village/area : _______________________

House number : _______________________

Name of the family head : _______________________

Age : _______________________

Sex : _______________________

Educational status : _______________________

Occupational status : _______________________

Address : _______________________

Common cooking method : Steaming/boiling/deep or shallow frying

Preparation of food : Hygienic/unhygienic

Commonly consuming food items : _______________________

 : _______________________

Particulars of Parents

Sl. No.	Name of the parents	Age	Sex	Education	Occupation	Remarks
1.						
2.						

Number of Living Children

Sl. No.	Name of the children	Order of live birth	Date of birth	Age	Sex	Education
1.						
2.						
3.						

Anthropometric Measurements

Weight (kg) : _______________________

Height or length (cm) : _______________________

Head circumference (cm) : _______________________

Chest circumference (cm) : _______________________

Midarm circumference (cm) : _______________________

Degree of Malnutrition

Body Mass Index

Growth Chart

Twenty Four-hour Dietary Recall Survey

Name of the area : _______________________________

Taluk : _______________________________

District : _______________________________

Religion : _______________________________

Total number of family members : _______________________________

Family income : _______________________________

Family Characteristics

Sl. No.	Name	Age	Occupation			Vegetarian	Nonvegetarian
			Sedentary	Moderate	Hard		
1.							
2.							
3.							
4.							
5.							
6.							

Purchase of Raw Material and Their Expenditure Per Day

Items	How often purchasing?			Monthly	Seasonally	Quantity	Expenditure per day
	Daily	Biweekly	Weekly				
Cereals							
Pulses							
Milk							
Fruits							
Vegetables							
Jaggery							
Sugar							
Ghee							
Oil							
Eggs							
Meat							
Fish							

Shopping facilities : Market/village shop/sunday market/any other forms
Preservation of raw foods : Store room/kitchen/no store/living room
Preservation of cooked foods : Refrigerator/cupboard/kitchen
Fuel used for cooking : Cooking gas/electrical stove/firewood/kerosene stove

Do You Have

Vegetable garden : _______________________________

Fruit tree : _______________________________

Household Animals

Cow   :____

Buffalo   :____

Hen   :____

Goat   :____

Pig   :____

Nutrition Cycle of the Family

Items/days	Items in grams							Average daily intake	Category
	1	2	3	4	5	6	7		
Wheat									Cereals
Rice									
Jowar									
Bajara									
Other									
Toor dal									Pulses
Arhar									
Urad									
Moong									
Green gram									
Groundnuts									
Others									
Milk									Milk products
Curd									
Buttermilk									
Others									
Oil									Fats
Ghee									
Dalda									
Leafy vegetables									Vegetables
Root/tubers									
Others									
Tea									Beverages
Coffee									
Others									
Sugar									Sugar
Jaggery									
Meat									Nonvegetarian
Fish									
Egg									

Contd...

Contd...

Items/days	Items in grams							Average daily intake	Category
	1	2	3	4	5	6	7		
Banana									Fruits
Orange									
Papaya									
Pineapple									
Grapes									
Apple									
Guava									
Others									

Inference

____
____
____
____
____
____
____
____
____
____
____
____
____
____
____
____
____
____
____
____
____
____
____
____
____

WHO Recommended Nutritive Values for Commonly Used Food Items in India

Sl. No.	Food preparation	Quantity per serving	Weight per serving	Calories (kcal)	Protein (g)	Fat (g)	Carbohydrates (g)	Calcium (g)	Phosphorus (g)	Iron (mg)
Cereal and Millet Preparation										
Rice preparation										
1.	Plain rice	2 servings	504	595	11.9	0.9	134.8	0.02	0.2	11.9
2.	Sambar rice	1 serving	485	405	13.5	13.5	76.2	0.08	0.16	13.5
3.	Curd rice	1 serving	253	221	6	7	33.3	0.57	0.10	6
4.	Sweet rice	1 serving	177	432	3.6	12	77.4	0.01	0.05	3.6
5.	Idli	2 pcs	136	130	4.6	0.2	27.6	0.03	0.08	4.6
6.	Plain dosa	2 pcs	100	216	4.1	9.7	28.2	0.03	0.07	4.1
7.	Masala dosa	2 pcs	100	212	4.6	8.4	29.4	0.04	0.08	4.6
8.	Pongal (hot)	1 serving	148	200	5.5	6	30.5	0.03	0.07	5.5
9.	Adai (hot)	1 pc	96	195	6.6	4.4	31.8	0.03	0.09	6.6
Wheat preparation										
1.	Wheat upma	1 serving	128	163	3.8	5.4	24.7	0.01	0.04	0.7
2.	Chapatis	2 pcs	57	196	5	5.5	30.8	0.13	0.02	3
3.	Puris	2 pcs	32	136	2.2	8.4	13	0.06	0.01	1.3
4.	Plain parathas	1 pc	66	104	4.5	19.6	27.3	0.12	0.01	2.7
5.	Rava dosa/Idli	2 pcs	114	212	5	8.5	28.7	0	0.06	0.9
6.	Kesari bath	1 serving	90	284	2	14.6	35.3	0.02	0.04	0.44
7.	Luchi	2 pcs	71	346	4	24	28	0.03	0.01	0.4
Millet preparation										
1.	Ragi balls	1 pc	336	446	6	7.6	86.8	0.3	0.4	6
2.	Ragi roti	2 pcs	185	460	8	9	87	0.3	0.4	6
3.	Maize roti	2 pcs	142	314	9.6	5.5	56.4	0.3	0.1	1.8
4.	Jowar roti	2 pcs	150	252	7.5	1.3	52.5	0.2	0.02	4.5
5.	Ragi puttu	1 plate	146	422	4.4	7.4	84	0.2	0.02	-
Pulse preparation										
1.	Bengal gram dal (cooked)	1½ cup	157	284	9	16.4	25.2	0.07	0.13	3.8
2.	Green gram dal (cooked)	1½ cup	142	171	7	7.7	18.4	0.08	0.09	2.7
3.	Red gram dal (cooked)	1½ cup	96	110	6.4	2	16.4	0.05	0.07	2.6
4.	Dal rasam	1½ cup	196	29	1.5	0.9	38	0.03	0.03	0.09
5.	Radish sambar (sundal)		196	101	4.1	3.6	13.1	0.04	0.07	2.2
6.	Green gram sambar (sundal)	1 plate	142	255	13.5	8.8	30.3	0.05	0.2	2.5
7.	Cowpea sundal	1 plate	142	259	13.1	9.2	30.9	0.08	0.2	4.8
8.	Amaranth sambar	1½ cup	140	250	5.1	2.7	13	0.05	0.08	8
9.	Bengal gram (sundal)	1 plate	142	272	13.2	11.1	29.7	0.11	0.15	5.5
Vegetable Preparation										
1.	Amaranth curry	1½ plate	28	47	1.4	2.3	5.1	0.04	0.04	6.64
2.	Amaranth masala	½ plate	42	46	1.2	2.6	44	0.05	0.05	6.8

Contd...

Contd...

Sl. No.	Food preparation	Quantity per serving	Weight per serving	Calories (kcal)	Protein (g)	Fat (g)	Carbohydrates (g)	Calcium (g)	Phospho-rus (g)	Iron (mg)
3.	Brinjal curry	½ plate	45	122	1.4	10.7	4.9	0.02	0.05	0.9
4.	Cabbage and carrot curry	½ plate	56	81	1.5	56	61	0.04	0.12	0.9
Egg, Milk, and Meat Preparation										
1.	Meat curry	1 serving	128	220	116	18	2.7	0.1	0.01	2.1
2.	Omelet	1 serving	39	77	5.8	5.7	0.5	0.03	0.1	1
3.	Meat fry	1 serving	142	339	21.8	26	4.5	0.23	0.2	3.3
4.	Fish fry	1 serving	100	220	16.2	16.2	1.4	0.05	0.45	1.2
5.	Rice, mutton pulav	2 servings	341	686	39	39	63.6	0.1	0.22	1.5
6.	Milk (buffalo)	1 cup	200	216	8.4	16	9.2	0.42	0.30	0.8
7.	Milk (cow)	1 cup	200	130	7	9.8	52.7	0.12	0.1	0.4
8.	Buttermilk	1 cup	200	36	1.8	2.8	4.8	0.07	0.07	0.2
9.	Buttermilk (buffalo)	1 cup	200	66	24	5.4	4.8	0.07	0.07	0.2
Preparation Containing Milk										
1.	Coffee	1 cup	200	104	3.8	3.4	14.4	0.1	0.1	1.2
2.	Tea	1 cup	200	72	1.4	1.6	13	0.06	0.04	-
3.	Cocoa	1 cup	200	174	7.5	20.2	20.2	0.2	0.15	0.3
4.	Wheat payasam	1 cup	154	178	3.4	31.5	31.5	0.09	0.08	0.4
5.	Rice payasam	1 cup	266	227	3.7	44.3	44.3	0.14	0.1	4.7
6.	Rice porridge	1 cup	280	263	7.6	44.7	35.9	0.3	0.2	0.7
7.	Bengal gram dal	1 cup	154	178	3.2	35.9	44.7	0.09	0.08	0.4
8.	Soy porridge	1 cup	154	178	7.7	44	44.7	0.07	0.14	0.4
9.	Wheat porridge	1 cup	280	263	7.6	44.7	35.9	0.3	0.22	0.7
10.	Ragi porridge	1 cup	193	317	8.7	52.7	35.9	0.24	0.22	1

7.6: Nutritional Assessment of Others

Identification Data

Name of the village/area : ____

House number : ____

Name of the family head : ____

Age : ____

Sex : ____

Educational status : ____

Occupational status : ____

Address : ____
____

Common cooking method : Steaming/boiling/deep or shallow frying

Preparation of food : Hygienic/unhygienic

Commonly consuming food items : ____
: ____

Particulars of Parents

Sl. No.	Name of the parents	Age	Sex	Education	Occupation	Remarks
1.						
2.						

Number of Living Children

Sl. No.	Name of the children	Order of live birth	Date of birth	Age	Sex	Education
1.						
2.						
3.						

Anthropometric Measurements

Weight (kg) : ____

Height or length (cm) : ____

Head circumference (cm) : ____

Chest circumference (cm) : ____

Midarm circumference (cm) : ____

Degree of Malnutrition

Body Mass Index

Growth Chart

Twenty Four-hour Dietary Recall Survey

Name of the area : _______________________________________

Taluk : _______________________________________

District : _______________________________________

Religion : _______________________________________

Total number of family members : _______________________________________

Family income : _______________________________________

Family Characteristics

| Sl. No. | Name | Age | Occupation | | | Vegetarian | Nonvegetarian |
			Sedentary	Moderate	Hard		
1.							
2.							
3.							
4.							
5.							
6.							

Purchase of Raw Material and Their Expenditure Per Day

| Items | How often purchasing? | | | Monthly | Seasonally | Quantity | Expenditure per day |
	Daily	Biweekly	Weekly				
Cereals							
Pulses							
Milk							
Fruits							
Vegetables							
Jaggery							
Sugar							
Ghee							
Oil							
Eggs							
Meat							
Fish							

Shopping facilities : Market/village shop/sunday market/any other forms

Preservation of raw foods : Store room/kitchen/no store/living room

Preservation of cooked foods : Refrigerator/cupboard/kitchen

Fuel used for cooking : Cooking gas/electrical stove/firewood/kerosene stove

Do You Have

Vegetable garden : _______________________________________

Fruit tree : _______________________________________

Household Animals

Cow : ____

Buffalo : ____

Hen : ____

Goat : ____

Pig : ____

Nutrition Cycle of the Family

Items/days	Items in grams							Average daily intake	Category
	1	2	3	4	5	6	7		
Wheat									Cereals
Rice									
Jowar									
Bajara									
Other									
Toor dal									Pulses
Arhar									
Urad									
Moong									
Green gram									
Groundnuts									
Others									
Milk									Milk products
Curd									
Buttermilk									
Others									
Oil									Fats
Ghee									
Dalda									
Leafy vegetables									Vegetables
Root/tubers									
Others									
Tea									Beverages
Coffee									
Others									
Sugar									Sugar
Jaggery									
Meat									Nonvegetarian
Fish									
Egg									

Contd...

Contd...

Items/days	Items in grams							Average daily intake	Category
	1	2	3	4	5	6	7		
Banana									Fruits
Orange									
Papaya									
Pineapple									
Grapes									
Apple									
Guava									
Others									

Inference

____
____
____
____
____
____
____
____
____
____
____
____
____
____
____
____
____
____
____
____
____
____
____
____

WHO Recommended Nutritive Values for Commonly Used Food Items in India

Sl. No.	Food preparation	Quantity per serving	Weight per serving	Calories (kcal)	Protein (g)	Fat (g)	Carbohydrates (g)	Calcium (g)	Phospho-rus (g)	Iron (mg)
Cereal and Millet Preparation										
Rice preparation										
1.	Plain rice	2 servings	504	595	11.9	0.9	134.8	0.02	0.2	11.9
2.	Sambar rice	1 serving	485	405	13.5	13.5	76.2	0.08	0.16	13.5
3.	Curd rice	1 serving	253	221	6	7	33.3	0.57	0.10	6
4.	Sweet rice	1 serving	177	432	3.6	12	77.4	0.01	0.05	3.6
5.	Idli	2 pcs	136	130	4.6	0.2	27.6	0.03	0.08	4.6
6.	Plain dosa	2 pcs	100	216	4.1	9.7	28.2	0.03	0.07	4.1
7.	Masala dosa	2 pcs	100	212	4.6	8.4	29.4	0.04	0.08	4.6
8.	Pongal (hot)	1 serving	148	200	5.5	6	30.5	0.03	0.07	5.5
9.	Adai (hot)	1 pc	96	195	6.6	4.4	31.8	0.03	0.09	6.6
Wheat preparation										
1.	Wheat upma	1 serving	128	163	3.8	5.4	24.7	0.01	0.04	0.7
2.	Chapatis	2 pcs	57	196	5	5.5	30.8	0.13	0.02	3
3.	Puris	2 pcs	32	136	2.2	8.4	13	0.06	0.01	1.3
4.	Plain parathas	1 pc	66	104	4.5	19.6	27.3	0.12	0.01	2.7
5.	Rava dosa/Idli	2 pcs	114	212	5	8.5	28.7	0	0.06	0.9
6.	Kesari bath	1 serving	90	284	2	14.6	35.3	0.02	0.04	0.44
7.	Luchi	2 pcs	71	346	4	24	28	0.03	0.01	0.4
Millet preparation										
1.	Ragi balls	1 pc	336	446	6	7.6	86.8	0.3	0.4	6
2.	Ragi roti	2 pcs	185	460	8	9	87	0.3	0.4	6
3.	Maize roti	2 pcs	142	314	9.6	5.5	56.4	0.3	0.1	1.8
4.	Jowar roti	2 pcs	150	252	7.5	1.3	52.5	0.2	0.02	4.5
5.	Ragi puttu	1 plate	146	422	4.4	7.4	84	0.2	0.02	-
Pulse preparation										
1.	Bengal gram dal (cooked)	1½ cup	157	284	9	16.4	25.2	0.07	0.13	3.8
2.	Green gram dal (cooked)	1½ cup	142	171	7	7.7	18.4	0.08	0.09	2.7
3.	Red gram dal (cooked)	1½ cup	96	110	6.4	2	16.4	0.05	0.07	2.6
4.	Dal rasam	1½ cup	196	29	1.5	09	38	0.03	0.03	0.09
5.	Radish sambar (sundal)		196	101	4.1	3.6	13.1	0.04	0.07	2.2
6.	Green gram sambar (sundal)	1 plate	142	255	13.5	8.8	30.3	0.05	0.2	2.5
7.	Cowpea sundal	1 plate	142	259	13 1	9.2	30.9	0.08	0.2	4.8
8.	Amaranth sambar	1½ cup	140	250	5.1	2.7	13	0.05	0.08	8
9.	Bengal gram (sundal)	1 plate	142	272	13.2	11.1	29.7	0.11	0.15	5.5
Vegetable Preparation										
1.	Amaranth curry	1½ plate	28	47	1.4	2.3	5.1	0.04	0.04	6.64
2.	Amaranth masala	½ plate	42	46	1.2	2.6	44	0.05	0.05	6.8

Contd...

Contd...

Sl. No.	Food preparation	Quantity per serving	Weight per serving	Calories (kcal)	Protein (g)	Fat (g)	Carbohydrates (g)	Calcium (g)	Phosphorus (g)	Iron (mg)
3.	Brinjal curry	½ plate	45	122	1.4	10.7	4.9	0.02	0.05	0.9
4.	Cabbage and carrot curry	½ plate	56	81	1.5	56	61	0.04	0.12	0.9
Egg, Milk, and Meat Preparation										
1.	Meat curry	1 serving	128	220	116	18	2.7	0.1	0.01	2.1
2.	Omelet	1 serving	39	77	5.8	5.7	0.5	0.03	0.1	1
3.	Meat fry	1 serving	142	339	21.8	26	4.5	0.23	0.2	3.3
4.	Fish fry	1 serving	100	220	16.2	16.2	1.4	0.05	0.45	1.2
5.	Rice, mutton pulav	2 servings	341	686	39	39	63.6	0.1	0.22	1.5
6.	Milk (buffalo)	1 cup	200	216	8.4	16	9.2	0.42	0.30	0.8
7.	Milk (cow)	1 cup	200	130	7	9.8	52.7	0.12	0.1	0.4
8.	Buttermilk	1 cup	200	36	1.8	2.8	4.8	0.07	0.07	0.2
9.	Buttermilk (buffalo)	1 cup	200	66	24	5.4	4.8	0.07	0.07	0.2
Preparation Containing Milk										
1.	Coffee	1 cup	200	104	3.8	3.4	14.4	0.1	0.1	1.2
2.	Tea	1 cup	200	72	1.4	1.6	13	0.06	0.04	-
3.	Cocoa	1 cup	200	174	7.5	20.2	20.2	0.2	0.15	0.3
4.	Wheat payasam	1 cup	154	178	3.4	31.5	31.5	0.09	0.08	0.4
5.	Rice payasam	1 cup	266	227	3.7	44.3	44.3	0.14	0.1	4.7
6.	Rice porridge	1 cup	280	263	7.6	44.7	35.9	0.3	0.2	0.7
7.	Bengal gram dal	1 cup	154	178	3.2	35.9	44.7	0.09	0.08	0.4
8.	Soy porridge	1 cup	154	178	7.7	44	44.7	0.07	0.14	0.4
9.	Wheat porridge	1 cup	280	263	7.6	44.7	35.9	0.3	0.22	0.7
10.	Ragi porridge	1 cup	193	317	8.7	52.7	35.9	0.24	0.22	1

7.7: Cooking Demonstration – 1

Introduction

Purpose of Demonstration

Method of Cooking

NUTRITIVE VALUES

Nutritional values of food

Items	Nutrient content	Amount of content	Nutrient value	Total values of calories

WHO recommended nutritive values for commonly used food items in India

Sl. No.	Food preparation	Quantity per serving	Weight per serving	Calories (kcal)	Protein (g)	Fat (g)	Carbohydrates (g)	Calcium (g)	Phosphorus (g)	Iron (mg)
Cereal and Millet Preparation										
Rice preparation										
1.	Plain rice	2 servings	504	595	11.9	0.9	134.8	0.02	0.2	11.9
2.	Sambar rice	1 serving	485	405	13.5	13.5	76.2	0.08	0.16	13.5
3.	Curd rice	1 serving	253	221	6	7	33.3	0.57	0.10	6
4.	Sweet rice	1 serving	177	432	3.6	12	77.4	0.01	0.05	3.6
5.	Idli	2 pcs	136	130	4.6	0.2	27.6	0.03	0.08	4.6
6.	Plain dosa	2 pcs	100	216	4.1	9.7	28.2	0.03	0.07	4.1
7.	Masala dosa	2 pcs	100	212	4.6	8.4	29.4	0.04	0.08	4.6
8.	Pongal (hot)	1 serving	148	200	5.5	6	30.5	0.03	0.07	5.5
9.	Adai (hot)	1 pc	96	195	6.6	4.4	31.8	0.03	0.09	6.6

Contd...

Contd...

Sl. No.	Food preparation	Quantity per serving	Weight per serving	Calories (kcal)	Protein (g)	Fat (g)	Carbohydrates (g)	Calcium (g)	Phospho-rus (g)	Iron (mg)
Wheat preparation										
1.	Wheat upma	1 serving	128	163	3.8	5.4	24.7	0.01	0.04	0.7
2.	Chapatis	2 pcs	57	196	5	5.5	30.8	0.13	0.02	3
3.	Puris	2 pcs	32	136	2.2	8.4	13	0.06	0.01	1.3
4.	Plain parathas	1 pc	66	104	4.5	19.6	27.3	0.12	0.01	2.7
5.	Rava dosa/Idli	2 pcs	114	212	5	8.5	28.7	0	0.06	0.9
6.	Kesari bath	1 serving	90	284	2	14.6	35.3	0.02	0.04	0.44
7.	Luchi	2 pcs	71	346	4	24	28	0.03	0.01	0.4
Millet preparation										
1.	Ragi balls	1 pc	336	446	6	7.6	86.8	0.3	0.4	6
2.	Ragi roti	2 pcs	185	460	8	9	87	0.3	0.4	6
3.	Maize roti	2 pcs	142	314	9.6	5.5	56.4	0.3	0.1	1.8
4.	Jowar roti	2 pcs	150	252	7.5	1.3	52.5	0.2	0.02	4.5
5.	Ragi puttu	1 plate	146	422	4.4	7.4	84	0.2	0.02	-
Pulse preparation										
1.	Bengal gram dal (cooked)	1½ cup	157	284	9	16.4	25.2	0.07	0.13	3.8
2.	Green gram dal (cooked)	1½ cup	142	171	7	7.7	18.4	0.08	0.09	2.7
3.	Red gram dal (cooked)	1½ cup	96	110	6.4	2	16.4	0.05	0.07	2.6
4.	Dal rasam	1½ cup	196	29	1.5	09	38	0.03	0.03	0.09
5.	Radish sambar (sundal)		196	101	4.1	3.6	13.1	0.04	0.07	2.2
6.	Green gram sambar (sundal)	1 plate	142	255	13.5	8.8	30.3	0.05	0.2	2.5
7.	Cowpea sundal	1 plate	142	259	13 1	9.2	30.9	0.08	0.2	4.8
8.	Amaranth sambar	1½ cup	140	250	5.1	2.7	13	0.05	0.08	8
9.	Bengal gram (sundal)	1 plate	142	272	13.2	11.1	29.7	0.11	0.15	5.5
Vegetable Preparation										
1.	Amaranth curry	1½ plate	28	47	1.4	2.3	5.1	0.04	0.04	6.64
2.	Amaranth masala	½ plate	42	46	1.2	2.6	44	0.05	0.05	6.8
3.	Brinjal curry	½ plate	45	122	1.4	10.7	4.9	0.02	0.05	0.9
4.	Cabbage and carrot curry	½ plate	56	81	1.5	56	61	0.04	0.12	0.9
Egg, Milk, and Meat Preparation										
1.	Meat curry	1 serving	128	220	116	18	2.7	0.1	0.01	2.1
2.	Omelet	1 serving	39	77	5.8	5.7	0.5	0.03	0.1	1
3.	Meat fry	1 serving	142	339	21.8	26	4.5	0.23	0.2	3.3
4.	Fish fry	1 serving	100	220	16.2	16.2	1.4	0.05	0.45	1.2
5.	Rice, mutton pulav	2 servings	341	686	39	39	63.6	0.1	0.22	1.5
6.	Milk (buffalo)	1 cup	200	216	8.4	16	9.2	0.42	0.30	0.8
7.	Milk (cow)	1 cup	200	130	7	9.8	52.7	0.12	0.1	0.4

Contd...

Contd...

Sl. No.	Food preparation	Quantity per serving	Weight per serving	Calories (kcal)	Protein (g)	Fat (g)	Carbohydrates (g)	Calcium (g)	Phosphorus (g)	Iron (mg)
8.	Buttermilk	1 cup	200	36	1.8	2.8	4.8	0.07	0.07	0.2
9.	Buttermilk (buffalo)	1 cup	200	66	24	5.4	4.8	0.07	0.07	0.2
Preparation Containing Milk										
1.	Coffee	1 cup	200	104	3.8	3.4	14.4	0.1	0.1	1.2
2.	Tea	1 cup	200	72	1.4	1.6	13	0.06	0.04	-
3.	Cocoa	1 cup	200	174	7.5	20.2	20.2	0.2	0.15	0.3
4.	Wheat payasam	1 cup	154	178	3.4	31.5	31.5	0.09	0.08	0.4
5.	Rice payasam	1 cup	266	227	3.7	44.3	44.3	0.14	0.1	4.7
6.	Rice porridge	1 cup	280	263	7.6	44.7	35.9	0.3	0.2	0.7
7.	Bengal gram dal	1 cup	154	178	3.2	35.9	44.7	0.09	0.08	0.4
8.	Soy porridge	1 cup	154	178	7.7	44	44.7	0.07	0.14	0.4
9.	Wheat porridge	1 cup	280	263	7.6	44.7	35.9	0.3	0.22	0.7
10.	Ragi porridge	1 cup	193	317	8.7	52.7	35.9	0.24	0.22	1

Health Education

Health education regarding importance of nutrition

| Time | Goals/objectives | Activities | | Audiovisual (AV) aids | Method of teaching | Evaluation |
		Teacher	Client			

Contd...

Contd...

Time	Goals/objectives	Activities		Audiovisual (AV) aids	Method of teaching	Evaluation
		Teacher	Client			

Evaluation for Cooking Demonstration

Name of the student   : ____

Batch (year)   : ____

Name of the recipient   : ____

Communication area   : ____

Date and time   : ____

Sl. No.	Criteria	Marks allotted	Marks obtained
1.	Required item to be selected according to the needs of recipient	2	
2.	Prepared and summated on the time	2	
3.	Assessment of nutrition status of family	2	
4.	Family members' interest	2	
5.	Way of preparation (hygiene, neat manner)	2	
6.	Selection of place and vessels	2	
7.	Way of serving	2	
8.	Cost-benefit	2	
9.	Calculation of nutritive values for food items	2	
10.	Feedback from the family members	2	
	Total	20	

Signature of the Student
Date:

Signature of the Clinical Coordinator
Date:

Signature of the HOD of Community Health Nursing
Date:

Cooking Demonstration – 2

Introduction

Purpose of Demonstration

Method of Cooking

NUTRITIVE VALUES

Nutritional Values of food

Items	Nutrient content	Amount of content	Nutrient value	Total values of calories

WHO Recommended Nutritive Values for Commonly Used Food Items in India

Sl. No.	Food preparation	Quantity per serving	Weight per serving	Calories (kcal)	Protein (g)	Fat (g)	Carbohydrates (g)	Calcium (g)	Phospho-rus (g)	Iron (mg)
Cereal and Millet Preparation										
Rice preparation										
1.	Plain rice	2 servings	504	595	11.9	0.9	134.8	0.02	0.2	11.9
2.	Sambar rice	1 serving	485	405	13.5	13.5	76.2	0.08	0.16	13.5
3.	Curd rice	1 serving	253	221	6	7	33.3	0.57	0.10	6
4.	Sweet rice	1 serving	177	432	3.6	12	77.4	0.01	0.05	3.6
5.	Idli	2 pcs	136	130	4.6	0.2	27.6	0.03	0.08	4.6
6.	Plain dosa	2 pcs	100	216	4.1	9.7	28.2	0.03	0.07	4.1
7.	Masala dosa	2 pcs	100	212	4.6	8.4	29.4	0.04	0.08	4.6
8.	Pongal (hot)	1 serving	148	200	5.5	6	30.5	0.03	0.07	5.5
9.	Adai (hot)	1 pc	96	195	6.6	4.4	31.8	0.03	0.09	6.6

Contd...

Contd...

Sl. No.	Food preparation	Quantity per serving	Weight per serving	Calories (kcal)	Protein (g)	Fat (g)	Carbohydrates (g)	Calcium (g)	Phosphorus (g)	Iron (mg)
Wheat preparation										
1.	Wheat upma	1 serving	128	163	3.8	5.4	24.7	0.01	0.04	0.7
2.	Chapatis	2 pcs	57	196	5	5.5	30.8	0.13	0.02	3
3.	Puris	2 pcs	32	136	2.2	8.4	13	0.06	0.01	1.3
4.	Plain parathas	1 pc	66	104	4.5	19.6	27.3	0.12	0.01	2.7
5.	Rava dosa/Idli	2 pcs	114	212	5	8.5	28.7	0	0.06	0.9
6.	Kesari bath	1 serving	90	284	2	14.6	35.3	0.02	0.04	0.44
7.	Luchi	2 pcs	71	346	4	24	28	0.03	0.01	0.4
Millet preparation										
1.	Ragi balls	1 pc	336	446	6	7.6	86.8	0.3	0.4	6
2.	Ragi roti	2 pcs	185	460	8	9	87	0.3	0.4	6
3.	Maize roti	2 pcs	142	314	9.6	5.5	56.4	0.3	0.1	1.8
4.	Jowar roti	2 pcs	150	252	7.5	1.3	52.5	0.2	0.02	4.5
5.	Ragi puttu	1 plate	146	422	4.4	7.4	84	0.2	0.02	-
Pulse preparation										
1.	Bengal gram dal (cooked)	1½ cup	157	284	9	16.4	25.2	0.07	0.13	3.8
2.	Green gram dal (cooked)	1½ cup	142	171	7	7.7	18.4	0.08	0.09	2.7
3.	Red gram dal (cooked)	1½ cup	96	110	6.4	2	16.4	0.05	0.07	2.6
4.	Dal rasam	1½ cup	196	29	1.5	09	38	0.03	0.03	0.09
5.	Radish sambar (sundal)		196	101	4.1	3.6	13.1	0.04	0.07	2.2
6.	Green gram sambar (sundal)	1 plate	142	255	13.5	8.8	30.3	0.05	0.2	2.5
7.	Cowpea sundal	1 plate	142	259	13 1	9.2	30.9	0.08	0.2	4.8
8.	Amaranth sambar	1½ cup	140	250	5.1	2.7	13	0.05	0.08	8
9.	Bengal gram (sundal)	1 plate	142	272	13.2	11.1	29.7	0.11	0.15	5.5
Vegetable Preparation										
1.	Amaranth curry	1½ plate	28	47	1.4	2.3	5.1	0.04	0.04	6.64
2.	Amaranth masala	½ plate	42	46	1.2	2.6	44	0.05	0.05	6.8
3.	Brinjal curry	½ plate	45	122	1.4	10.7	4.9	0.02	0.05	0.9
4.	Cabbage and carrot curry	½ plate	56	81	1.5	56	61	0.04	0.12	0.9
Egg, Milk, and Meat Preparation										
1.	Meat curry	1 serving	128	220	116	18	2.7	0.1	0.01	2.1
2.	Omelet	1 serving	39	77	5.8	5.7	0.5	0.03	0.1	1
3.	Meat fry	1 serving	142	339	21.8	26	4.5	0.23	0.2	3.3
4.	Fish fry	1 serving	100	220	16.2	16.2	1.4	0.05	0.45	1.2
5.	Rice, mutton pulav	2 servings	341	686	39	39	63.6	0.1	0.22	1.5
6.	Milk (buffalo)	1 cup	200	216	8.4	16	9.2	0.42	0.30	0.8
7.	Milk (cow)	1 cup	200	130	7	9.8	52.7	0.12	0.1	0.4

Contd...

Contd...

Sl. No.	Food preparation	Quantity per serving	Weight per serving	Calories (kcal)	Protein (g)	Fat (g)	Carbohydrates (g)	Calcium (g)	Phospho-rus (g)	Iron (mg)
8.	Buttermilk	1 cup	200	36	1.8	2.8	4.8	0.07	0.07	0.2
9.	Buttermilk (buffalo)	1 cup	200	66	24	5.4	4.8	0.07	0.07	0.2
Preparation Containing Milk										
1.	Coffee	1 cup	200	104	3.8	3.4	14.4	0.1	0.1	1.2
2.	Tea	1 cup	200	72	1.4	1.6	13	0.06	0.04	-
3.	Cocoa	1 cup	200	174	7.5	20.2	20.2	0.2	0.15	0.3
4.	Wheat payasam	1 cup	154	178	3.4	31.5	31.5	0.09	0.08	0.4
5.	Rice payasam	1 cup	266	227	3.7	44.3	44.3	0.14	0.1	4.7
6.	Rice porridge	1 cup	280	263	7.6	44.7	35.9	0.3	0.2	0.7
7.	Bengal gram dal	1 cup	154	178	3.2	35.9	44.7	0.09	0.08	0.4
8.	Soy porridge	1 cup	154	178	7.7	44	44.7	0.07	0.14	0.4
9.	Wheat porridge	1 cup	280	263	7.6	44.7	35.9	0.3	0.22	0.7
10.	Ragi porridge	1 cup	193	317	8.7	52.7	35.9	0.24	0.22	1

Health Education

Health education regarding importance of nutrition

Time	Goals/objectives	Activities		Audiovisual (AV) aids	Method of teaching	Evaluation
		Teacher	Client			

Contd...

Contd...

| Time | Goals/objectives | Activities | | Audiovisual (AV) aids | Method of teaching | Evaluation |
		Teacher	Client			

Evaluation for Cooking Demonstration

Name of the student   : _______________________________

Batch (year)   : _______________________________

Name of the recipient   : _______________________________

Communication area   : _______________________________

Date and time   : _______________________________

Sl. No.	Criteria	Marks allotted	Marks obtained
1.	Required item to be selected according to the needs of recipient	2	
2.	Prepared and summated on the time	2	
3.	Assessment of nutrition status of family	2	
4.	Family members' interest	2	
5.	Way of preparation (hygiene, neat manner)	2	
6.	Selection of place and vessels	2	
7.	Way of serving	2	
8.	Cost-benefit	2	
9.	Calculation of nutritive values for food items	2	
10.	Feedback from the family members	2	
	Total	20	

Signature of the Student   **Signature of the Clinical Coordinator**

Date: **Date:**

Signature of the HOD of Community Health Nursing

Date:

8.1: Water Purification Site

Introduction

Objectives of Water Purification

Disinfectant Agent

Aims of Water Purification

Steps of Water Purification (Name of Water Purification Center) _______________________

Staffing Pattern

Laboratory Test Report

Conclusion

Signature of the Clinical Instructor

Date:

Signature of HOD of Community Health Nursing

Date:

8.2: Milk Diary

Introduction

Objectives of Milk Diary

Definition

Raw Milk, Collection, Conception

Separation and Storage, Standardization

Homogenization

Milk Production

Type of Milk

Products

Packing of Milk

Cream Separation

Cleaning Procedure

Staffing Pattern

Conclusion

____

____

____

____

____

____

Signature of the Clinical Instructor

Date:

Signature of HOD of Community Health Nursing

Date:

8.3: Slaughter House

Introduction

Slaughter House

a. Stock area

b. Slaughter area

Function of Slaughter House

Conclusion

Signature of the Clinical Instructor   **Signature of HOD of Community Health Nursing**

Date: **Date:**

8.4: Sewage Disposable Site

Introduction

____

____

____

____

____

____

Methods

____

____

____

____

____

____

Function

____

____

____

____

____

____

Conclusion

____

____

____

____

____

____

Signature of the Clinical Instructor   **Signature of HOD of Community Health Nursing**

Date: Date:

8.5: Rainwater Harvesting

Introduction

Definition of Water Cycle

Needs for Rainwater Harvesting

Way of Collection Harvesting Rainwater

Storage of Rainwater and Uses

Conclusion

Signature of the Clinical Instructor

Signature of HOD of Community Health Nursing

Date:

Date:

8.6: Market

Introduction

Types of Market

Collection and Storage of Materials

Disposal of Waste Material

Conclusion

____

____

____

____

____

____

Signature of the Clinical Instructor

Signature of HOD of Community Health Nursing

Date:

Date:

9.1: Health Education/Counseling

Identification Data

Name of the student : ____
Topic : ____
Method of teaching : ____
Audiovisual aids : ____
Duration : ____
Place : ____
Date : ____
Focus group : ____

Needs of Education

____

____

____

____

____

____

____

____

____

Objectives of Education

____

____

____

____

____

____

____

____

____

Health Education Regarding Importance of Nutrition

Time	Goals/objectives	Activities		Audiovisual (AV) aids	Method of teaching	Evaluation
		Teacher	Client			

Contd...

Contd...

Time	Goals/objectives	Activities		Audiovisual (AV) aids	Method of teaching	Evaluation
		Teacher	**Client**			

Contd...

Contd...

Time	Goals/objectives	Activities		Audiovisual (AV) aids	Method of teaching	Evaluation
		Teacher	Client			

Contd...

Contd...

Time	Goals/objectives	Activities		Audiovisual (AV) aids	Method of teaching	Evaluation
		Teacher	Client			

Contd...

Contd...

Time	Goals/objectives	Activities		Audiovisual (AV) aids	Method of teaching	Evaluation
		Teacher	Client			

Evaluation Proforma for Health Education

Name of the student   :____

Date and time   :____

Topic   :____

Community area   :____

Name of the clinical instructor :____

Sl. No.	Criteria	Excellent 5	Very good 4	Average 3	Poor 2	Very poor 1
1.	**Content:** • Relevant • Adequate • Organization • Depth of knowledge • Recent advancement					
2.	**Presentation:** • Voice audible • Clarity • Modulation • Confidence • Posture language • Motivated • Group participation • Feedback					
3.	**Audiovisual aids:** • Appropriate • Preparation • Visibility • Proper usage • Follow principles • Replace of material • Time management					
	Total					
	Comments					

Signature of the Clinical Instructor   **Signature of the HOD of Community Health Nursing**

Date: **Date:**

10.1: Charts

Introduction

Objectives of Charts

Principles of Charts

Types of Charts

Method of Preparation

How to Use the Chart

Conclusion

10.2: Diorama

Introduction

Objectives of Diorama

Principles of Diorama

Method of Preparation

Conclusion

10.3: Flannel Graphs

Introduction

Objectives of Flannel Graphs

Principles of Flannel Graphs

Method of Preparation

Conclusion

____

____

____

____

____

____

____

10.4: Flash Card

Introduction

Objectives of Flash Card

Principles of Flash Card

Method of Preparation

Conclusion

10.5: Flip Chart

Introduction

Objectives of Flip Chart

Principles of Flip Chart

Method of Preparation

Conclusion

10.6: Pamphlet/Leaflet

Introduction

Objectives of Pamphlet/Leaflet

Principles of Pamphlet/Leaflet

Method of Preparation

Conclusion

10.7: Posters

Introduction

Objectives of Posters

Principles of Posters

Method of Preparation

**Conclusion

FAMILY CARE PLAN (RURAL) – 1

Identification Data

House number   : _______________________________

Name of the informer   : _______________________________

Age   : _______________________________

Sex   : _______________________________

Name of the head of the family   : _______________________________

Address   : _______________________________

____

____

____

____

Type of family   : _______________________________

Family size   : _______________________________

Religion   : _______________________________

Caste   : _______________________________

Educational status   : _______________________________

Occupational status   : _______________________________

Income of the family   : ₹ ___________________________/month

Mother tongue   : _______________________________

Student Data

Name of the student   : _______________________________

Course   : _______________________________

Class   : _______________________________

Date of care started   : _______________________________

Date of care ended   : _______________________________

Family Composition

Sl. No.	Name of the family members	Age	Sex	Relationship with head of the family	Educational status	Occupational status	Health status
1.							
2.							
3.							
4.							
5.							
6.							
7.							

Socioeconomic Status

____

____

____

Family Tree

Past Medical History

Past Surgical History

Present History of Illness

Housing Pattern (Floor Map)

Housing and Environmental Condition

Type of house		
Roof	:	Thatch/thatti/tilled/terraced/others
Floor	:	Mud/tiled/cemented/others
Wall	:	Thatti/mud/brick/cement plastered/others
Housing pattern	:	Pucca/semi pucca/kutcha/others
Possession	:	Own house/rental house/leased
Area (square feet)	:	Adequate/inadequate
Ventilation	:	Natural/artificial
Number of rooms	:	
Doors/windows	:	Adequate/inadequate
Electricity	:	Available/not available
Mode of lighting	:	Oil lamp/kerosene/electric bulb/others
Water supply	:	Adequate/inadequate
Mode of water supply	:	Well/public tap/hand pump/others
Latrine	:	Service/water seal/open field
Drain	:	Open/closed/nil
Street light	:	Yes/No
Street road condition	:	Cement/tar/mud/others
Type of fuel used	:	Firewood/kerosene/gas/cow dung/biogas
Open space around the house	:	Yes/No
Garden	:	Yes/No
Water stagnation	:	Yes/No
Disposal of waste	:	Drum/open space/manure pit/burning/throwing into street/separate
Livestock and poultry	:	Available/not available
If available	:	Shed/separate
	:	Attached/mixed
Healthcare facilities	:	GH/PHC/SC/private doctors/others
Medical aid available in the street	:	Doctor/homeo/siddha/village Vaidyas/others
Playground in the street	:	Available/not available
Social institution	:	Bank/post office/police station/market/transport
Educational institution	:	Primary school/secondary school/HSS/college/night school/adult school/crèche
Religious institution	:	Temple/church/mosque/others
Presence of rodents	:	
Presence of stray dog	:	
Presence of domestic animals	:	
Presence of insects	:	

Economical Status

Income   : _________________________ per month

Source of income   : _________________________

Number of earning members : _________________________

Expenditure   : _________________________ per month

Rent   : _________________________ per month

Food   : _________________________ per month

Health   : _________________________ per month

School   : _________________________ per month

Miscellaneous   : _________________________ per month

Own properties   : _________________________ Land/vehicle/house

Transportation

Bus   : _________________________ Specify, which bus: _________________________

Auto rickshaw   : _________________________ Yes/No

Four wheelers   : _________________________ Yes/No

Train   : _________________________ Yes/No

Airway   : _________________________ Yes/No

Communication

Face-to-face   : _________________________

Mobile   : _________________________

Telephone   : _________________________

Through letter   : _________________________

Internet   : _________________________

Personal Hobbies

Recreational activity : _________________________

Nutritional Status of Family

Dietary pattern   : Vegetarian/nonvegetarian/ovo vegetarian

Frequency of nonvegetarian : _________________________

Food habit: Number of meals : _________________________ /day

Cooking method   : _________________________

Staple food   : _________________________

Sources of food items

(vegetables)   : _________________________

Storage of food items : _________________________

Usage of processed food items : _________________________

Menu Plan

Sl. No.	Type of food	Amount of food	Calories (kcal)
Breakfast			
1.			
2.			
Midmorning			
1.			
2.			
Lunch			
1.			
2.			
3.			
Evening			
1.			
2.			
Dinner			
1.			
2.			
3.			
Total			

Amount allotted for nutrition : _______________________

Use of vegetables : _______________________

Fruits : _______________________

Cereals/pulses/nuts : _______________________

Beneficiary Data

Name of beneficiary : _______________________

Age : _______________________

Sex : _______________________

Plan for Home Visit

Sl. No.	Name of the beneficiary	Date	Needs/problems	Preventions	Short-term goals	Long-term goals
1.						
2.						

Physical Examination

General appearance
Nourishment : ____
Body built : ____
Health : ____
Activity : ____

Mental status
Consciousness : ____
Look : ____

Vital signs
Temperature : ____
Pulse : ____
Respiration : ____
Blood pressure : ____

Anthropometric measurement
Height or length (cm) : ____
Weight (kg) : ____
Chest circumference (cm) : ____
Midarm circumference (cm) : ____
Body mass index (BMI) : ____
Skin condition : ____
Color : ____
Texture : ____
Lesion : ____
Sensation : ____

Head and face
Scalp : ____
Face : ____
Color of hair : ____

Eyes
Eyebrows : ____
Eyelashes : ____
Eyelids : ____
Eyeball : ____
Conjunctiva : ____
Lens : ____
Vision : ____

Nose
External nose : ____
Nostrils : ____
Nasal septum : ____
Sinuses ____

Ears
External ear : ____
Tympanic membrane : ____
Hearing acuity : ____

Mouth
Lips : ____
Odors : ____
Teeth : ____
Tongue : ____
Speech : ____

Neck
**Thyroid gland and lymph
node enlargement**

Inspection : _______________________________

____

____

____

Palpation : _______________________________

____

____

____

Chest

Inspection : _______________________________
Palpation : _______________________________
Percussion : _______________________________
Auscultation : _______________________________

Abdomen

Inspection : _______________________________
Palpation : _______________________________
Auscultation : _______________________________
Percussion : _______________________________

Genitalia

____

____

Back (vertebral column) : Mention any abnormal posturing/lordosis/scoliosis/kyphosis
Impression : _______________________________
Extremities : Present/absent
If any illness, specify : _______________________________

List of Nursing Diagnosis

1. _______________________________

2. _______________________________

3. _______________________________

4. _______________________________

5. _______________________________

6. _______________________________

Nursing Care Plan

Assessment of the problems	Nursing diagnosis	Goals/objectives	Interventions	Implementation	Rationales	Evaluation

Contd...

Contd...

Assessment of the problems	Nursing diagnosis	Goals/objectives	Interventions	Implementation	Rationales	Evaluation

Contd...

Contd...

Assessment of the problems	Nursing diagnosis	Goals/objectives	Interventions	Implementation	Rationales	Evaluation

Contd...

Contd...

Assessment of the problems	Nursing diagnosis	Goals/objectives	Interventions	Implementation	Rationales	Evaluation

Health Education

____
____
____
____
____
____

Nurses Report

Sl. No.	Date	Name of the beneficiary	Age	Sex	Problem	Procedure done	Remarks/ finding	Signature of the student
1.								
2.								

Conclusion

____
____
____
____
____
____
____

Signature of the Student
Date:

Signature of the Clinical Instructor
Date:

FAMILY CARE PLAN (URBAN) – 2

Identification Data

House number : ____
Name of the informer : ____
Age : ____
Sex : ____
Name of the head of the family : ____
Address : ____
____
____
____

Type of family : ____
Family size : ____
Religion : ____
Caste : ____
Educational status : ____
Occupational status : ____
Income of the family : ₹ ______________________________________/month
Mother tongue : ____

Student data

Name of the student : ____
Course : ____
Class : ____
Date of care started : ____
Date of care ended : ____

Family Composition

Sl. No.	Name of the family members	Age	Sex	Relationship with head of the family	Educational status	Occupational status	Health status
1.							
2.							
3.							
4.							
5.							
6.							
7.							

Socioeconomic Status

____

____

____

Family Tree

Past Medical History

____

____

____

____

____

Past Surgical History

____

____

____

____

____

Present History of Illness

____

____

____

____

____

Housing Pattern (Floor Map)

Housing and Environmental Condition

Type of house	
Roof	: Thatch/thatti/tilled/terraced/others
Floor	: Mud/tiled/cemented/others
Wall	: Thatti/mud/brick/cement plastered/others
Housing pattern	: Pucca/semi pucca/kutcha/others
Possession	: Own house/rental house/leased
Area (square feet)	: Adequate/inadequate
Ventilation	: Natural/artificial
Number of rooms	:
Doors/windows	: Adequate/inadequate
Electricity	: Available/not available
Mode of lighting	: Oil lamp/kerosene/electric bulb/others
Water supply	: Adequate/inadequate
Mode of water supply	: Well/public tap/hand pump/others
Latrine	: Service/water seal/open field
Drain	: Open/closed/nil
Street light	: Yes/No
Street road condition	: Cement/tar/mud/others
Type of fuel used	: Firewood/kerosene/gas/cow dung/biogas
Open space around the house	: Yes/No
Garden	: Yes/No
Water stagnation	: Yes/No
Disposal of waste	: Drum/open space/manure pit/burning/throwing into street/separate
Livestock and poultry	: Available/not available
If available	: Shed/separate : Attached/mixed
Healthcare facilities	: GH/PHC/SC/private doctors/others
Medical aid available in the street	: Doctor/homeo/siddha/village Vaidyas/others
Playground in the street	: Available/not available
Social institution	: Bank/post office/police station/market/transport
Educational institution	: Primary school/secondary school/HSS/college/night school/adult school/crèche
Religious institution	: Temple/church/mosque/others
Presence of rodents	:
Presence of stray dog	:
Presence of domestic animals	:
Presence of insects	:

Economical Status

Income   : _________________ per month
Source of income   : _________________
Number of earning members   : _________________
Expenditure   : _________________ per month
Rent   : _________________ per month
Food   : _________________ per month
Health   : _________________ per month
School   : _________________ per month
Miscellaneous   : _________________ per month
Own properties   : _________________ Land/vehicle/house

Transportation

Bus   : _________________ Specify, which bus: _________________
Auto rickshaw   : _________________ Yes/No
Four wheelers   : _________________ Yes/No
Train   : _________________ Yes/No
Airway   : _________________ Yes/No

Communication

Face-to-face   : _________________
Mobile   : _________________
Telephone   : _________________
Through letter   : _________________
Internet   : _________________

Personal Hobbies

Recreational activity   : _________________

Nutritional Status of Family

Dietary pattern   : Vegetarian/nonvegetarian/ovo vegetarian
Frequency of nonvegetarian   : _________________
Food habit: Number of meals   : _________________/day
Cooking method   : _________________
Staple food   : _________________
Sources of food items
(vegetables)   : _________________
Storage of food items   : _________________
Usage of processed food items   : _________________

Menu Plan

Sl. No.	Type of food	Amount of food	Calories (kcal)
Breakfast			
1.			
2.			
Midmorning			
1.			
2.			
Lunch			
1.			
2.			
3.			
Evening			
1.			
2.			
Dinner			
1.			
2.			
3.			
Total			

Amount allotted for nutrition : _______________________________________

Use of vegetables : _______________________________________

Fruits : _______________________________________

Cereals/pulses/nuts : _______________________________________

Beneficiary Data

Name of beneficiary : _______________________________________

Age : _______________________________________

Sex : _______________________________________

Plan for Home Visit

Sl. No.	Name of the beneficiary	Date	Needs/problems	Preventions	Short-term goals	Long-term goals
1.						
2.						

Physical Examination

General appearance

Nourishment : ____
Body built : ____
Health : ____
Activity : ____

Mental status

Consciousness : ____
Look : ____

Vital signs

Temperature : ____
Pulse : ____
Respiration : ____
Blood pressure : ____

Anthropometric measurement

Height or length (cm) : ____
Weight (kg) : ____
Chest circumference (cm) : ____
Midarm circumference (cm) : ____
Body mass index (BMI) : ____
Skin condition : ____
Color : ____
Texture : ____
Lesion : ____
Sensation : ____

Head and face

Scalp : ____
Face : ____
Color of hair : ____

Eyes

Eyebrows : ____
Eyelashes : ____
Eyelids : ____
Eyeball : ____
Conjunctiva : ____
Lens : ____
Vision : ____

Nose

External nose : ____
Nostrils : ____
Nasal septum : ____
Sinuses ____

Ears

External ear : ____
Tympanic membrane : ____
Hearing acuity : ____

Mouth

Lips : ____
Odors : ____
Teeth : ____
Tongue : ____
Speech : ____

Neck
Thyroid gland and lymph
node enlargement
Inspection   : ______________________________________
____
____
____

Palpation   : ______________________________________
____
____
____

Chest
Inspection   : ______________________________________
Palpation   : ______________________________________
Percussion   : ______________________________________
Auscultation   : ______________________________________
Abdomen
Inspection   : ______________________________________
Palpation   : ______________________________________
Auscultation   : ______________________________________
Percussion   : ______________________________________
Genitalia
____
____

Back (vertebral column)   : Mention any abnormal posturing/lordosis/scoliosis/kyphosis
Impression   : ______________________________________
Extremities   : Present/absent
If any illness, specify   : ______________________________________

List of Nursing Diagnosis

1. ____
2. ____
3. ____
4. ____
5. ____
6. ____

Nursing Care Plan

Assessment of the problems	Nursing diagnosis	Goals/objectives	Interventions	Implementation	Rationales	Evaluation

Contd...

Contd...

Assessment of the problems	Nursing diagnosis	Goals/objectives	Interventions	Implementation	Rationales	Evaluation

Contd...

Contd...

Assessment of the problems	Nursing diagnosis	Goals/objectives	Interventions	Implementation	Rationales	Evaluation

Contd...

Contd...

Assessment of the problems	Nursing diagnosis	Goals/objectives	Interventions	Implementation	Rationales	Evaluation

Health Education

____

____

____

____

____

____

Nurses Report

Sl. No.	Date	Name of the beneficiary	Age	Sex	Problem	Procedure done	Remarks/ finding	Signature of the student
1.								
2.								

Conclusion

____

____

____

____

____

____

____

Signature of the Student
Date:

Signature of the Clinical Instructor
Date:

FAMILY CARE PLAN – 3

Identification Data

House number : ______________________________
Name of the informer : ______________________________
Age : ______________________________
Sex : ______________________________
Name of the head of the family : ______________________________
Address : ______________________________
____
____

Type of family : ______________________________
Family size : ______________________________
Religion : ______________________________
Caste : ______________________________
Educational status : ______________________________
Occupational status : ______________________________
Income of the family : ₹ ______________________________/month
Mother tongue : ______________________________

Student Data

Name of the student : ______________________________
Course : ______________________________
Class : ______________________________
Date of care started : ______________________________
Date of care ended : ______________________________

Family Composition

Sl. No.	Name of the family members	Age	Sex	Relationship with head of the family	Educational status	Occupational status	Health status
1.							
2.							
3.							
4.							
5.							
6.							
7.							

Socioeconomic Status

____

____

____

Family Tree

Past Medical History

____
____
____
____
____
____

Past Surgical History

____
____
____
____
____
____

Present History of Illness

____
____
____
____
____
____

Housing Pattern (Floor Map)

Housing and Environmental Condition

Type of house	
Roof	: Thatch/thatti/tilled/terraced/others
Floor	: Mud/tiled/cemented/others
Wall	: Thatti/mud/brick/cement plastered/others
Housing pattern	: Pucca/semi pucca/kutcha/others
Possession	: Own house/rental house/leased
Area (square feet)	: Adequate/inadequate
Ventilation	: Natural/artificial
Number of rooms	:
Doors/windows	: Adequate/inadequate
Electricity	: Available/not available
Mode of lighting	: Oil lamp/kerosene/electric bulb/others
Water supply	: Adequate/inadequate
Mode of water supply	: Well/public tap/hand pump/others
Latrine	: Service/water seal/open field
Drain	: Open/closed/nil
Street light	: Yes/No
Street road condition	: Cement/tar/mud/others
Type of fuel used	: Firewood/kerosene/gas/cow dung/biogas
Open space around the house	: Yes/No
Garden	: Yes/No
Water stagnation	: Yes/No
Disposal of waste	: Drum/open space/manure pit/burning/throwing into street/separate
Livestock and poultry	: Available/not available
If available	: Shed/separate : Attached/mixed
Healthcare facilities	: GH/PHC/SC/private doctors/others
Medical aid available in the street	: Doctor/homeo/siddha/village Vaidyas/others
Playground in the street	: Available/not available
Social institution	: Bank/post office/police station/market/transport
Educational institution	: Primary school/secondary school/HSS/college/night school/adult school/crèche
Religious institution	: Temple/church/mosque/others
Presence of rodents	:
Presence of stray dog	:
Presence of domestic animals	:
Presence of insects	:

Economical Status

Income   : _________________ per month

Source of income   : _________________

Number of earning members   : _________________

Expenditure   : _________________ per month

Rent   : _________________ per month

Food   : _________________ per month

Health   : _________________ per month

School   : _________________ per month

Miscellaneous   : _________________ per month

Own properties   : _________________ Land/vehicle/house

Transportation

Bus   : _________________ Specify, which bus: _________________

Auto rickshaw   : _________________ Yes/No

Four wheelers   : _________________ Yes/No

Train   : _________________ Yes/No

Airway   : _________________ Yes/No

Communication

Face-to-face   : ____

Mobile   : ____

Telephone   : ____

Through letter   : ____

Internet   : ____

Personal Hobbies

Recreational activity   : ____

Nutritional Status of Family

Dietary pattern   : Vegetarian/nonvegetarian/ovo vegetarian

Frequency of nonvegetarian   : ____

Food habit: Number of meals   : _____________________________________/day

Cooking method   : ____

Staple food   : ____

Sources of food items

(vegetables)   : ____

Storage of food items   : ____

Usage of processed food items : ____

Menu Plan

Sl. No.	Type of food	Amount of food	Calories (kcal)
Breakfast			
1.			
2.			
Midmorning			
1.			
2.			
Lunch			
1.			
2.			
3.			
Evening			
1.			
2.			
Dinner			
1.			
2.			
3.			
Total			

Amount allotted for nutrition : _______________________

Use of vegetables : _______________________

Fruits : _______________________

Cereals/pulses/nuts : _______________________

Beneficiary Data

Name of beneficiary : _______________________

Age : _______________________

Sex : _______________________

Plan for Home Visit

Sl. No.	Name of the beneficiary	Date	Needs/problems	Preventions	Short-term goals	Long-term goals
1.						
2.						

Physical Examination

General appearance
Nourishment : _______________________
Body built : _______________________
Health : _______________________
Activity : _______________________

Mental status
Consciousness : _______________________
Look : _______________________

Vital signs
Temperature : _______________________
Pulse : _______________________
Respiration : _______________________
Blood pressure : _______________________

Anthropometric measurement
Height or length (cm) : _______________________
Weight (kg) : _______________________
Chest circumference (cm) : _______________________
Midarm circumference (cm) : _______________________
Body mass index (BMI) : _______________________
Skin condition : _______________________
Color : _______________________
Texture : _______________________
Lesion : _______________________
Sensation : _______________________

Head and face
Scalp : _______________________
Face : _______________________
Color of hair : _______________________

Eyes
Eyebrows : _______________________
Eyelashes : _______________________
Eyelids : _______________________
Eyeball : _______________________
Conjunctiva : _______________________
Lens : _______________________
Vision : _______________________

Nose
External nose : _______________________
Nostrils : _______________________
Nasal septum : _______________________
Sinuses _______________________

Ears
External ear : _______________________
Tympanic membrane : _______________________
Hearing acuity : _______________________

Mouth
Lips : _______________________
Odors : _______________________
Teeth : _______________________
Tongue : _______________________
Speech : _______________________

Neck
Thyroid gland and lymph
node enlargement

Inspection   : _______________________________

____

____

____

Palpation   : _______________________________

____

____

____

Chest
Inspection   : _______________________________
Palpation   : _______________________________
Percussion   : _______________________________
Auscultation   : _______________________________

Abdomen
Inspection   : _______________________________
Palpation   : _______________________________
Auscultation   : _______________________________
Percussion   : _______________________________

Genitalia

____

____

Back (vertebral column) : Mention any abnormal posturing/lordosis/scoliosis/kyphosis

Impression   : _______________________________

Extremities   : Present/absent

If any illness, specify : _______________________________

List of Nursing Diagnosis

1. _______________________________

2. _______________________________

3. _______________________________

4. _______________________________

5. _______________________________

6. _______________________________

Nursing Care Plan

Assessment of the problems	Nursing diagnosis	Goals/objectives	Interventions	Implementation	Rationales	Evaluation

Contd...

Contd...

Assessment of the problems	Nursing diagnosis	Goals/objectives	Interventions	Implementation	Rationales	Evaluation

Contd...

Contd...

Assessment of the problems	Nursing diagnosis	Goals/objectives	Interventions	Implementation	Rationales	Evaluation

Contd...

Contd...

Assessment of the problems	Nursing diagnosis	Goals/objectives	Interventions	Implementation	Rationales	Evaluation

Health Education

____

____

____

____

____

____

Nurses Report

Sl. No.	Date	Name of the beneficiary	Age	Sex	Problem	Procedure done	Remarks/ finding	Signature of the student
1.								
2.								

Conclusion

____

____

____

____

____

____

____

Signature of the Student
Date:

Signature of the Clinical Instructor
Date:

FAMILY CARE STUDY (RURAL)

Identification Data

House number   : ____

Name of the informer   : ____

Age   : ____

Sex   : ____

Name of the head of the family   : ____

Address   : ____

____

____

____

Type of family   : ____

Family size   : ____

Religion   : ____

Caste   : ____

Educational status   : ____

Occupational status   : ____

Income of the family   : _______________________________/month

Mother tongue   : ____

Student Data

Name of the student   : ____

Course   : ____

Class   : ____

Date of care started   : ____

Date of care ended   : ____

Family Composition

Sl. No.	Name of the family members	Age	Sex	Relationship with head of the family	Educational status	Occupational status	Health status
1.							
2.							
3.							
4.							
5.							
6.							
7.							

Socioeconomic Status

____

____

____

Family Tree

Past Medical History

Past Surgical History

Present History of Illness

Housing Pattern (Floor Map)

Housing and Environmental Condition

Type of house		
	Roof	: Thatch/thatti/tilled/terraced/others
	Floor	: Mud/tiled/cemented/others
	Wall	: Thatti/mud/brick/cement plastered/others
	Housing pattern	: Pucca/semi pucca/kutcha/others
	Possession	: Own house/rental house/leased
Area (square feet)		: Adequate/inadequate
Ventilation		: Natural/artificial
Number of rooms		:
Doors/windows		: Adequate/inadequate
Electricity		: Available/not available
	Mode of lighting	: Oil lamp/kerosene/electric bulb/others
Water supply		: Adequate/inadequate
Mode of water supply		: Well/public tap/hand pump/others
Latrine		: Service/water seal/open field
Drain		: Open/closed/nil
Street light		: Yes/No
Street road condition		: Cement/tar/mud/others
Type of fuel used		: Firewood/kerosene/gas/cow dung/biogas
Open space around the house		: Yes/No
Garden		: Yes/No
Water stagnation		: Yes/No
Disposal of waste		: Drum/open space/manure pit/burning/throwing into street/separate
Livestock and poultry		: Available/not available
	If available	: Shed/separate : Attached/mixed
Healthcare facilities		: GH/PHC/SC/private doctors/others
Medical aid available in the street		: Doctor/homeo/siddha/village vaidyas/others
Playground in the street		: Available/not available
Social institution		: Bank/post office/police station/market/transport
Educational institution		: Primary school/secondary school/HSS/college/night school/adult school/crèche
Religious institution		: Temple/church/mosque/others
Presence of rodents		:
Presence of stray dog		:
Presence of domestic animals		:
Presence of insects		:

Economical Status

Income : ________________________ per month

Source of income : ________________________

Number of earning members : ________________________

Expenditure : ________________________ per month

Rent : ________________________ per month

Food : ________________________ per month

Health : ________________________ per month

School : ________________________ per month

Miscellaneous : ________________________ per month

Own properties : ________________________ Land/vehicle/house

Transportation

Bus : ________________________ Specify, which bus: __________

Auto rickshaw : ________________________ Yes/No

Four wheelers : ________________________ Yes/No

Train : ________________________ Yes/No

Airway : ________________________ Yes/No

Communication

Face-to-face : ________________________

Mobile : ________________________

Telephone : ________________________

Through letter : ________________________

Internet : ________________________

Personal hobbies

Recreational activity : ________________________

Nutritional Status of Family

Dietary pattern : Vegetarian/nonvegetarian/ovo vegetarian

Frequency of nonvegetarian : ________________________

Food habit: Number of meals : ________________________/day

Cooking method : ________________________

Staple food : ________________________

Sources of food items

(vegetables) : ________________________

Storage of food items : ________________________

Usage of processed food items : ________________________

Menu Plan

Sl. No.	Type of food	Amount of food	Calories (kcal)
Breakfast			
1.			
2.			
Midmorning			
1.			
2.			
Lunch			
1.			
2.			
3.			
Evening			
1.			
2.			
Dinner			
1.			
2.			
3.			
Total			

Amount allotted for nutrition : ______________________________

Use of vegetables : ______________________________

Fruits : ______________________________

Cereals/pulses/nuts : ______________________________

Plan for Home Visit

Sl. No.	Name of the beneficiary	Date	Needs/problems	Preventions	Short-term goals	Long-term goals
1.						
2.						

Cooking Demonstration

____
____
____
____
____
____
____
____

Beneficiary Data

Name of beneficiary   : ____
Age   : ____
Sex   : ____

Plan for Home Visit

Sl. No.	Name of the beneficiary	Date	Needs/problems	Preventions	Short-term goals	Long-term goals
1.						
2.						

Physical Examination

General appearance

Nourishment   : ____
Body built   : ____
Health   : ____
Activity   : ____

Mental status

Consciousness : ____
Look   : ____

Vital signs

Temperature   : ____
Pulse   : ____
Respiration   : ____
Blood pressure : ____

Anthropometric measurement

Height or length (cm)   : ____
Weight (kg)   : ____
Chest circumference (cm)   : ____
Midarm circumference (cm) : ____
Body mass index (BMI)   : ____
Skin condition   : ____
Color   : ____
Texture   : ____
Lesion   : ____
Sensation   : ____

Head and face

Scalp   : ____
Face   : ____
Color of hair : ____

Eyes

Eyebrows   : ____
Eyelashes : ____
Eyelids   : ____
Eyeball   : ____

Conjunctiva : __________________________
Lens : __________________________
Vision : __________________________

Nose
External nose : __________________________
Nostrils : __________________________
Nasal septum : __________________________
Sinuses : __________________________

Ears
External ear : __________________________
Tympanic membrane : __________________________
Hearing acuity : __________________________

Mouth
Lips : __________________________
Odors : __________________________
Teeth : __________________________
Tongue : __________________________
Speech : __________________________

Neck
Thyroid gland and lymph node enlargement
Inspection : __________________________
____
____
____

Palpation : __________________________
____
____
____

Chest
Inspection : __________________________
Palpation : __________________________
Percussion : __________________________
Auscultation : __________________________

Abdomen
Inspection : __________________________
Palpation : __________________________
Auscultation : __________________________
Percussion : __________________________

Genitalia
____
____

Back (vertebral column) : Mention any abnormal posturing/lordosis/scoliosis/kyphosis
Impression : __________________________
Extremities : Present/absent
If any illness, specify : __________________________

Investigation

Sl. No.	Investigation	Normal value	Patient value	Remarks
1.				
2.				
3.				
4.				
5.				
6.				
7.				

Medication

Sl. No.	Medication	Route/amount	Action	Side effect	Remarks
1.					
2.					
3.					
4.					
5.					

Book Picture

Nursing Diagnosis

1. ____
2. ____
3. ____
4. ____
5. ____
6. ____

Nursing Care Plan

Assessment of the problems	Nursing diagnosis	Goals/objectives	Interventions	Implementation	Rationales	Evaluation

Contd...

Contd...

Assessment of the problems	Nursing diagnosis	Goals/objectives	Interventions	Implementation	Rationales	Evaluation

Contd...

Contd...

Assessment of the problems	Nursing diagnosis	Goals/objectives	Interventions	Implementation	Rationales	Evaluation

Contd...

Contd...

Assessment of the problems	Nursing diagnosis	Goals/objectives	Interventions	Implementation	Rationales	Evaluation

Note: In assessment column, subjective data and objective data should be included.

Health Education

____
____
____
____
____
____

Nurses Report

Sl. No.	Date	Name of the beneficiary	Age	Sex	Problem	Procedure done	Remarks/ finding	Signature of the student
1.								
2.								

Conclusion

____
____
____
____
____
____
____

Bibliography

____
____
____
____
____
____
____
____

Signature of the Student
Date:

Signature of the Clinical Instructor
Date:

FAMILY CARE STUDY (URBAN)

Identification Data

House number   : ____

Name of the informer   : ____

Age   : ____

Sex   : ____

Name of the head of the family   : ____

Address   : ____

____

____

____

Type of family   : ____

Family size   : ____

Religion   : ____

Caste   : ____

Educational status   : ____

Occupational status   : ____

Income of the family   : ____/month

Mother tongue   : ____

Student Data

Name of the student   : ____

Course   : ____

Class   : ____

Date of care started   : ____

Date of care ended   : ____

Family Composition

Sl. No.	Name of the family members	Age	Sex	Relationship with head of the family	Educational status	Occupational status	Health status
1.							
2.							
3.							
4.							
5.							
6.							
7.							

Socioeconomic Status

____

____

____

____

Family Tree

Past Medical History

Past Surgical History

Present History of Illness

Housing Pattern (Floor Map)

Housing and Environmental Condition

Type of house		
	Roof	: Thatch/thatti/tilled/terraced/others
	Floor	: Mud/tiled/cemented/others
	Wall	: Thatti/mud/brick/cement plastered/others
	Housing pattern	: Pucca/semi pucca/kutcha/others
	Possession	: Own house/rental house/leased
Area (square feet)		: Adequate/inadequate
Ventilation		: Natural/artificial
Number of rooms		:
Doors/windows		: Adequate/inadequate
Electricity		: Available/not available
	Mode of lighting	: Oil lamp/kerosene/electric bulb/others
Water supply		: Adequate/inadequate
	Mode of water supply	: Well/public tap/hand pump/others
Latrine		: Service/water seal/open field
Drain		: Open/closed/nil
Street light		: Yes/No
Street road condition		: Cement/tar/mud/others
Type of fuel used		: Firewood/kerosene/gas/cow dung/biogas
Open space around the house		: Yes/No
Garden		: Yes/No
Water stagnation		: Yes/No
Disposal of waste		: Drum/open space/manure pit/burning/throwing into street/separate
Livestock and poultry		: Available/not available
	If available	: Shed/separate : Attached/mixed
Healthcare facilities		: GH/PHC/SC/private doctors/others
Medical aid available in the street		: Doctor/homeo/siddha/village vaidyas/others
Playground in the street		: Available/not available
Social institution		: Bank/post office/police station/market/transport
Educational institution		: Primary school/secondary school/HSS/college/night school/adult school/crèche
Religious institution		: Temple/church/mosque/others
Presence of rodents		:
Presence of stray dog		:
Presence of domestic animals		:
Presence of insects		:

Economical Status

Income   : ________________________ per month

Source of income   : ________________________

Number of earning members   : ________________________

Expenditure   : ________________________ per month

Rent   : ________________________ per month

Food   : ________________________ per month

Health   : ________________________ per month

School   : ________________________ per month

Miscellaneous   : ________________________ per month

Own properties   : ________________________ Land/vehicle/house

Transportation

Bus   : ________________________ Specify, which bus : __________

Auto rickshaw   : ________________________ Yes/No

Four wheelers   : ________________________ Yes/No

Train   : ________________________ Yes/No

Airway   : ________________________ Yes/No

Communication

Face-to-face   : ____

Mobile   : ____

Telephone   : ____

Through letter   : ____

Internet   : ____

Personal hobbies

Recreational activity   : ____

Nutritional Status of Family

Dietary pattern   : Vegetarian/nonvegetarian/ov ovegetarian

Frequency of nonvegetarian   : ____

Food habit: Number of meals   : ______________________________________/day

Cooking method   : ____

Staple food   : ____

Sources of food items
(vegetables)   : ____

 Storage of food items   : ____

Usage of processed food items   : ____

Menu Plan

Sl. No.	Type of food	Amount of food	Calories (kcal)
Breakfast			
1.			
2.			
Midmorning			
1.			
2.			
Lunch			
1.			
2.			
3.			
Evening			
1.			
2.			
Dinner			
1.			
2.			
3.			
Total			

Amount allotted for nutrition : ____

Use of vegetables : ____

Fruits : ____

Cereals/pulses/nuts : ____

Plan for Home Visit

Sl. No.	Name of the beneficiary	Date	Needs/problems	Preventions	Short-term goals	Long-term goals
1.						
2.						

Cooking Demonstration

____

____

____

____

____

____

Beneficiary Data

Name of beneficiary : _______________________________

Age : _______________________________

Sex : _______________________________

Plan for Home Visit

Sl. No.	Name of the beneficiary	Date	Needs/problems	Preventions	Short-term goals	Long-term goals
1.						
2.						

Physical Examination

General appearance

Nourishment : _______________________________

Body built : _______________________________

Health : _______________________________

Activity : _______________________________

Mental status

Consciousness : _______________________________

Look : _______________________________

Vital signs

Temperature : _______________________________

Pulse : _______________________________

Respiration : _______________________________

Blood pressure : _______________________________

Anthropometric measurement

Height or length (cm) : _______________________________

Weight (kg) : _______________________________

Chest circumference (cm) : _______________________________

Midarm circumference (cm) : _______________________________

Body mass index (BMI) : _______________________________

Skin condition : _______________________________

Color : _______________________________

Texture : _______________________________

Lesion : _______________________________

Sensation : _______________________________

Head and face

Scalp : _______________________________

Face : _______________________________

Color of hair : _______________________________

Eyes

Eyebrows : _______________________________

Eyelashes : _______________________________

Eyelids : _______________________________

Eyeball	: _______________________
Conjunctiva	: _______________________
Lens	: _______________________
Vision	: _______________________

Nose

External nose	: _______________________
Nostrils	: _______________________
Nasal septum	: _______________________
Sinuses	: _______________________

Ears

External ear	: _______________________
Tympanic membrane	: _______________________
Hearing acuity	: _______________________

Mouth

Lips	: _______________________
Odors	: _______________________
Teeth	: _______________________
Tongue	: _______________________
Speech	: _______________________

Neck

Thyroid gland and lymph node enlargement

Inspection : _______________________

Palpation : _______________________

Chest

Inspection	: _______________________
Palpation	: _______________________
Percussion	: _______________________
Auscultation	: _______________________

Abdomen

Inspection	: _______________________
Palpation	: _______________________
Auscultation	: _______________________
Percussion	: _______________________

Genitalia

Back (vertebral column) : Mention any abnormal posturing/lordosis/scoliosis/kyphosis

Impression : _______________________

Extremities : Present/absent

If any illness, specify : _______________________

Investigation

Sl. No.	Investigation	Normal value	Patient value	Remarks
1.				
2.				
3.				
4.				
5.				
6.				
7.				

Medication

Sl. No.	Medication	Route/amount	Action	Side effect	Remarks
1.					
2.					
3.					
4.					
5.					

Book Picture

Nursing Diagnosis

1.
2.
3.
4.
5.
6.

Nursing Care Plan

Assessment of the problems	Nursing diagnosis	Goals/objectives	Interventions	Implementation	Rationales	Evaluation

Contd...

Contd...

Assessment of the problems	Nursing diagnosis	Goals/objectives	Interventions	Implementation	Rationales	Evaluation

Contd...

Contd...

Assessment of the problems	Nursing diagnosis	Goals/objectives	Interventions	Implementation	Rationales	Evaluation

Contd...

Contd...

Assessment of the problems	Nursing diagnosis	Goals/objectives	Interventions	Implementation	Rationales	Evaluation

Note: In assessment column, subjective data and objective data should be included.

Health Education

____
____
____
____
____

Nurses Report

Sl. No.	Date	Name of the beneficiary	Age	Sex	Problem	Procedure done	Remarks/ finding	Signature of the student
1.								
2.								

Conclusion

____
____
____
____
____
____
____
____

Bibliography

____
____
____
____
____
____
____
____

Signature of the Student
Date:

Signature of the Clinical Instructor
Date:

Identification Data

Name   : ____

Relationship with head of family   : ____

Self/wife/son/daughter/any other   : ____

Age   : ____

Religion   : ____

Education   : ____

Occupation   : ____

Monthly income   : ____

Gender: Male/female   : ____

Marital status   : ____

Address   : ____

Contact No.   : ____

Name of the Health Facility–DH/CHC/PHC/SC/.......   **Date:**

Checklist Biomedical Waste Management–DH

Health facility/ward	Response		Remarks
Black bags	Yes	No	
Located at right place			
Placed on stand			
Contain only noninfected waste			
Is it torn?			
Available sufficiently			
Collected daily			
Yellow bags			
Located at right place			
Placed on stand			
Contain only infected waste			
Is it torn/leaking?			
Available sufficiently			
Collected daily			
Bleaching solution			
Is it prepared today?			
Separate bucket for needle/sharps and other plastic material Does the bucket contain mesh?			
Available in sufficient quantity?			
Is it covered properly?			
Needle destroyers			
Present			
Working			
Location is appropriate			
Syringes			
All syringes are in bucket for disinfection			
Collected daily			

Contd...

Contd...

Health facility/ward	Response			Remarks
Gloves				
Disposed in bleaching solution				
Available in sufficient quantity				
Available of appropriate size				
Housekeeping				
Floor hygiene	Good	OK	Poor	Bad
Toilets cleanliness	Good	OK	Poor	Bad

Comments

____
____
____
____
____
____
____
____
____
____
____
____
____
____
____
____
____
____
____
____
____
____

Signature: **Signature of the Academic Counselor/Supervisor**

Checklist for Biomedical Waste Management – CHC

Health facility/ward	Response		Remarks
Black bags	Yes	No	
Located at right place			
Placed on stand			
Contain only noninfected waste			
Is it torn?			
Available sufficiently			
Collected daily			
Yellow bags			
Located at right place			
Placed on stand			
Contain only infected waste			
Is it torn/leaking?			
Available sufficiently			
Collected daily			
Bleaching solution			
Is it prepared today?			
Separate bucket for needle/sharps and other plastic material Does the bucket contain mesh?			
Available in sufficient quantity?			
Is it covered properly?			
Needle destroyers			
Present			
Working			
Location is appropriate			
Syringes			
All syringes are in bucket for disinfection			
Collected daily			
Gloves			
Disposed in bleaching solution			

Contd...

Health facility/ward	Response			Remarks
Available in sufficient quantity				
Available of appropriate size				
Housekeeping				
Floor hygiene	Good	OK	Poor	Bad
Toilets cleanliness	Good	OK	Poor	Bad

Comments

Signature: **Signature of the Academic Counselor/Supervisor**

14. RECORDS AND REPORTS

Visit and observe the Health Facilities of Records and Registers maintain and findings after completing the various activates given below:

Name of the Health Centre   : ____

Date   : ____

Map of the community:

Identify the village to be covered for preparing map:

Activities of Records:

Sl. No.	Content/Steps	Finding and Remarks

Signature of the Student   **Signature of the Supervisor**

Date: **Date:**

Signature of the HOD of Community Health Nursing

Date:

Identification Data

Name of the area rural/urban : _______________________________________

House No. : _______________________________________

Name of the health center : _______________________________________

Name of the head of the family : _______________________________________

Family identification : _______________________________________

Total No. of members in the family : _______________________________________

Type of family: Nuclear/non-nuclear :

Religion : Hindu: _____________ Muslim: _____________ Christian: _____________

Others : _______________________________________

Specify subcaste : _______________________________________

Language known : _______________________________________

Name of the informer : _______________________________________

Age/sex : _______________________________________

Address : _______________________________________

Education status : _______________________________________

Occupational status : _______________________________________

Income of the family : _____________________________________/month

Findings/diagnosis of the patient : _______________________________________

* Health personnel to be check signs and symptoms based on that treatment to decide.

Investigation of an Outbreak

Steps	Findings and reporting
Ensure existence of outbreak	
Confirm diagnosis with the help of authorized health professional. Estimate the number of cases	
Analyses then data in terms of time, place and person	
Determine who is at risk of contracting the diseases	
Prepare written report	

Sl. No.	Details	Findings	Management/referral
1.	Identification No:		
2.	Date and time:		
3.	Name:		
4.	Age:		
5.	Sex:		
6.	Address: Residence, workplace separately		
7.	Contact No:		
8.	Symptoms present, date and time of onset:		
9.	Source of water supply-tap/hand pump/well/river/ponds/natural water body/etc. History of travel outside/history of intake food items outside house, items taken/any medication taken and names/any laboratory investigations; check and note based on available records/family members list with age, sex, any family members suffering from the infection, their onset day and time.		

16.1: Identification of Appropriate Management of Communicable Disease

Identification Data

Name of the area rural/urban : _______________________________

House No. : _______________________________

Name of the health center : _______________________________

Name of the head of the family : _______________________________

Family identification : _______________________________

Total No. of members in the family : _______________________________

Type of family: Nuclear/non-nuclear : _______________________________

Religion : Hindu: __________ Muslim: __________ Christian: __________

Others : _______________________________

Specify subcaste : _______________________________

Language known : _______________________________

Name of the informer : _______________________________

Age/sex : _______________________________

Address : _______________________________

Educational status : _______________________________

Occupational status : _______________________________

Income of the family : ____________________________/month

Findings/diagnosis of the patient : _______________________________

** Health personnel to be check signs and symptoms based on that treatment to decide.*

Sl. No.	Communicable	Causes	Findings of causes	Management and referral services
1.	**Present history**			
2.	**Past history**			
3.	**Family history**			
4.	**Malaria**	Attacks of fever, every 3rd or 4th day with three stages		
5.	**Cold stage**	• Headache • Nausea • Vomiting • Chills with rigors		
6.	**Hot stage**	Headache worsens and temperature is very hot, lasts from 2–6 hours		
7.	**Sweating stage**	• Temperature drops down to normal with profuse sweating • Jaundice • Anemia		
8.	**Kala azar**	• Fever • Splenomegaly and hepatomegaly • Anemia • Weight loss • Darkening of skin of face hands, feet and abdomen • Lymphadenopathy multiple nodular infiltration of skin usually without ulceration • Painful ulcers in part of body exposed to send fly		
9.	**Japanese encephalitis (JE)**	Viral infection presents classical symptoms similar to any other viral encephalitis • Fever (38–41°C) • Headache • Meningitis • Encephalitis, severe rigors stupor • Disorientation • Coma • Tremors • Paralysis (generalized/hypertonia) loss of coordination, etc.		
10.	**Dengue fever**	Assess for flu-like symptoms which lasts for 2–7 days. High fever (40°C/104°F) is usually accompanied by at least two of the following symptoms: • Headache • Pain behind eyes • Nausea, vomiting • Swollen glands • Joint, bone or muscle pains • Rash		

Contd...

Contd...

Sl. No.	Communicable	Causes	Findings of causes	Management and referral services
11.	**Tuberculosis**	• A bad cough that lasts 3 weeks or longer • Pain in the chest • Coughing up blood or sputum (phlegm from deep inside the lungs) • Weakness or fatigue • Weight loss • No appetite • Chills • Fever • Sweating at night		
12.	**Leprosy**	• Discolored patches of **skin**, usually flat, that may be numb and look faded (lighter than the **skin** around) • Growths (**nodules**) on the **skin** • Thick, stiff or dry **skin** • Painless **ulcers** on the soles of feet • Painless **swelling** or **lumps** on the face or earlobes • **Loss** of eyebrows or eyelashes		
13.	**AIDS**	Rapid weight loss Recurring **fever** or profuse **night sweats** Extreme and unexplained **tiredness** Prolonged swelling of the **lymph glands** in the armpits, groin, or neck Diarrhea that lasts for more than a week Sores of the mouth, anus, or genitals Pneumonia		
14.	**Chickenpox**	The itchy blister rash caused by chickenpox infection appears 10 to 21 days after exposure to the virus and usually lasts about 5 to 10 days. Other signs and symptoms, which may appear 1 to 2 days before the rash, include: • Fever • Loss of appetite • Headache • Tiredness and a general feeling of being unwell (malaise) Once the chickenpox rash appears, it goes through three phases: 1. Raised pink or red bumps (papules), which break out over several days 2. Small fluid-filled blisters (vesicles), which form in about one day and then break and leak 3. Crusts and scabs, which cover the broken blisters and take several more days to heal		
15.	**Measles**	• Cough • Fever • Runny nose • Red eyes • Sore throat • White spots inside the mouth		
16.	**Mumps**	• Fatigue • Body aches • Headache • Loss of appetite • Low-grade fever		

Contd...

Contd...

Sl. No.	Communicable	Causes	Findings of causes	Management and referral services
17.	**Rubella**	<ul><li>A **low-grade fever**</li><li>**Headache**</li><li>Mild pink eye (redness or swelling of the white of the eye)</li><li>General discomfort</li><li>Swollen and **enlarged lymph nodes**</li><li>Cough</li><li>**Runny nose**</li></ul>		
18.	**Diphtheria**	A thick, gray membrane covering your throat and tonsils A **sore throat** and hoarseness **Swollen glands (enlarged lymph nodes)** in your **neck** **Difficulty breathing** or rapid breathing Nasal discharge Fever and chills		
19.	**Hepatitis**	<ul><li>Bile production, which is essential to digestion</li><li>Filtering of toxins from your body</li><li>Excretion of bilirubin (a product of broken-down red blood cells), cholesterol, hormones, and drugs</li><li>Breakdown of carbohydrates, fats, and proteins</li><li>Activation of enzymes, which are specialized proteins essential to body functions</li><li>Storage of glycogen (a form of sugar), minerals, and vitamins (A, D, E, and K)</li><li>Synthesis of blood proteins, such as albumin</li><li>Synthesis of clotting factors</li></ul>		
20.	**Poliomyelitis**	<ul><li>**Sore throat**</li><li>**Fever**</li><li>**Tiredness**</li><li>Nausea</li><li>**Headache**</li><li>Stomach pain</li></ul>		
21.	**COVID -19**	The most common symptoms of COVID-19 are:<ul><li>Fever</li><li>Dry cough</li><li>Fatigue</li></ul>Other symptoms that are less common and may affect some patients include:<ul><li>Loss of taste or smell</li><li>Nasal congestion</li><li>Conjunctivitis (also known as red eyes)</li><li>Sore throat</li><li>Headache</li><li>Muscle or joint pain</li><li>Different types of skin rash</li><li>Nausea or vomiting</li><li>Diarrhea</li><li>Chills or dizziness</li></ul>		

Signature of HOD/Clinical Instructor   **Signature of Principal**

16.2: Identification of Appropriate Management of Noncommunicable Diseases

IDENTIFICATION DATA

Name of the area rural/urban : _______________________________

House No. : _______________________________

Name of the health center : _______________________________

Name of the head of the family : _______________________________

Family identification : _______________________________

Total No. of members in the family : _______________________________

Type of family: Nuclear/non-nuclear : _______________________________

Religion : Hindu: _____________ Muslim: _____________ Christian: _____________

Others : _______________________________

Specify subcaste : _______________________________

Language known : _______________________________

Name of the informer : _______________________________

Age/sex : _______________________________

Address : _______________________________

Education status : _______________________________

Occupational status : _______________________________

Income of the family : _______________________________/month

Findings/diagnosis of the patient : _______________________________

Health personnel to be check signs and symptoms based on that treatment to decide.

Sl. No.	Noncommunicable	Causes	Findings of causes	Management and referral services
1.	**Cardiovascular disease (CVD)** Coronary heart disease	• Chest pain (angina) with sternal pressure radiation to the neck, jaw, arm with duration <20–30 minutes which may be associated with dyspnea • Palpitation, nausea and vomiting		
2.	**Myocardial infarction (MI)**	• Has angina increased intensity and duration >30 minutes. Associate symptoms: • Weakness • Nausea • Vomiting • Sweating • Apprehension • Anxiety • Sense of impending doom		
3.	**Stroke**	Sudden onset of the following: • Weakness of one half of body or one part of body • Inability or difficulty in speech • Imbalance • Blindness • Dizziness or spinning • Severe headache • Seizures • Loss of consciousness		
4.	**Uncontrolled hyperglycemia**	• Excess thirst • Excess urination • Excess hunger with loss of weight • Frequent infection • Nonhealing wounds		
5.	**Diabetic mellitus**	• Increased thirst • **Frequent urination** • Extreme **hunger** • Unexplained **weight loss** • Presence of ketones in the urine (ketones are a byproduct of the breakdown of muscle and fat that happens when there's not enough available insulin) • **Fatigue** • Irritability • Blurred vision		
6.	**Hypertension**	• Severe headaches • Nosebleed • Fatigue or confusion • Vision problems • Chest pain • **Difficulty breathing** • Irregular heartbeat • **Blood in the urine**		

Contd...

Contd...

Sl. No.	Noncommunicable	Causes	Findings of causes	Management and referral services
7.	**Cardiac diseases**	• **Chest pain, chest tightness, chest pressure** and **chest discomfort** (angina) • **Shortness of breath** • Pain, numbness, weakness or coldness in your legs or arms if the blood vessels in those parts of your body are narrowed • Pain in the neck, jaw, throat, upper abdomen or back		
8.	**Cancer**	• Persistent cough or blood-tinged saliva • A change in bowel habits • **Blood in the stool** • Unexplained anemia (low blood count) • **Breast lump** or breast discharge • Lumps in the testicles • A change in urination		
9.	**Renal disorder**	• Weight loss and poor appetite • Swollen **ankles, feet** or hands—as a result of water retention (edema) • Shortness of breath • **Tiredness** • Blood in your pee **(urine)** • An increased need to pee—particularly at night • Difficulty sleeping (insomnia) • Itchy skin		

Signature of HOD/Clinical Instructor   **Signature of Principal**

17.1: BAG TECHNIQUE PROCEDURE – 1

Identification Data

Name of the student   : _______________________________________

Name of the procedure   : _______________________________________

Date of the procedure   : _______________________________________

Name of the patient   : _______________________________________

House number   : _______________________________________

Age of the patient   : _______________________________________

Sex of the patient   : _______________________________________

Education of the patient   : _______________________________________

Occupation of the patient   : _______________________________________

Requirement of the procedure : _______________________________________

Name of the supervisor   : _______________________________________

Nursing Diagnosis of the Patient

____

____

____

____

____

____

____

Objectives of the Procedure

____

____

____

____

____

____

____

Requirement of Articles

Initial Preparation of Patient

Procedure

Health Education About Procedure

Conclusion

Checklist for Bag Technique Procedure

Sl. No.	Knowledge and skills	Marks allotted	Score obtained by the student
1.	Essential supplies and equipment	2	
2.	Explain the procedure to the patient	2	
3.	Spreading of newspaper	2	
4.	Way of opening the bag	2	
5.	Handling of handwashing articles	2	
6.	Handwashing techniques	3	
7.	Handling necessary articles for the procedure	2	
8.	Maintain comfortable position of the patient	2	
9.	Maintain good communication skills and knowledge	2	
10.	Performing the procedure	4	
11.	Discharge the waste	2	
12.	Replacement of the articles	2	
13.	Folding the newspapers	2	
14.	Wash hands and close the bag	2	
15.	Knowledge about the usage of the bag	2	
16.	Record the result	1	
17.	Report to the clinical instructor (supervisor)	1	
	Total marks	35	

Signature of the Student

Date:

Signature of the Supervisor

Date:

Signature of the HOD of Community Health Nursing

Date:

BAG TECHNIQUE PROCEDURE – 2

Identification Data

Name of the student : _______________________________

Name of the procedure : _______________________________

Date of the procedure : _______________________________

Name of the patient : _______________________________

House number : _______________________________

Age of the patient : _______________________________

Sex of the patient : _______________________________

Education of the patient : _______________________________

Occupation of the patient : _______________________________

Requirement of the procedure : _______________________________

Name of the supervisor : _______________________________

Nursing Diagnosis of the Patient

Objectives of the Procedure

Requirement of Articles

Initial Preparation of Patient

Procedure

Health Education About Procedure

Conclusion

Checklist for Bag Technique Procedure

Sl. No.	Knowledge and skills	Marks allotted	Score obtained by the student
1.	Essential supplies and equipment	2	
2.	Explain the procedure to the patient	2	
3.	Spreading of newspaper	2	
4.	Way of opening the bag	2	
5.	Handling of handwashing articles	2	
6.	Handwashing techniques	3	
7.	Handling necessary articles for the procedure	2	
8.	Maintain comfortable position of the patient	2	
9.	Maintain good communication skills and knowledge	2	
10.	Performing the procedure	4	
11.	Discharge the waste	2	
12.	Replacement of the articles	2	
13.	Folding the newspapers	2	
14.	Wash hands and close the bag	2	
15.	Knowledge about the usage of the bag	2	
16.	Record the result	1	
17.	Report to the clinical instructor (supervisor)	1	
	Total marks	**35**	

Signature of the Student

Date:

Signature of the Supervisor

Date:

Signature of the HOD of Community Health Nursing

Date:

BAG TECHNIQUE PROCEDURE – 3

Identification Data

Name of the student : ___________________________

Name of the procedure : ___________________________

Date of the procedure : ___________________________

Name of the patient : ___________________________

House number : ___________________________

Age of the patient : ___________________________

Sex of the patient : ___________________________

Education of the patient : ___________________________

Occupation of the patient : ___________________________

Requirement of the procedure : ___________________________

Name of the supervisor : ___________________________

Nursing Diagnosis of the Patient

Objectives of the Procedure

Requirement of Articles

Initial Preparation of Patient

Procedure

Health Education About Procedure

Conclusion

Checklist for Bag Technique Procedure

Sl. No.	Knowledge and skills	Marks allotted	Score obtained by the student
1.	Essential supplies and equipment	2	
2.	Explain the procedure to the patient	2	
3.	Spreading of newspaper	2	
4.	Way of opening the bag	2	
5.	Handling of handwashing articles	2	
6.	Handwashing techniques	3	
7.	Handling necessary articles for the procedure	2	
8.	Maintain comfortable position of the patient	2	
9.	Maintain good communication skills and knowledge	2	
10.	Performing the procedure	4	
11.	Discharge the waste	2	
12.	Replacement of the articles	2	
13.	Folding the newspapers	2	
14.	Wash hands and close the bag	2	
15.	Knowledge about the usage of the bag	2	
16.	Record the result	1	
17.	Report to the clinical instructor (supervisor)	1	
	Total marks	35	

Signature of the Student

Date:

Signature of the Supervisor

Date:

Signature of the HOD of Community Health Nursing

Date:

17.2: Hand Washing Skills

Identification Data

Name	: _______________________________
Relationship with head of family	: _______________________________
Self/wife/son/daughter/any other	: _______________________________
Age	: _______________________________
Religion	: _______________________________
Education	: _______________________________
Occupation	: _______________________________
Monthly income	: _______________________________
Gender: Male/female:	: _______________________________
Marital status	: _______________________________
	: _______________________________
	: _______________________________
	: _______________________________
Address	: _______________________________
Contact No.	: _______________________________

Six steps of hand washing are shown in figure
- Step 1: Palm to palm
- Step 2: Back of both hand
- Step 3: In between the finger
- Step 4: Back of the fingers
- Step 5: The thumbs
- Step 6: Tip of the fingers

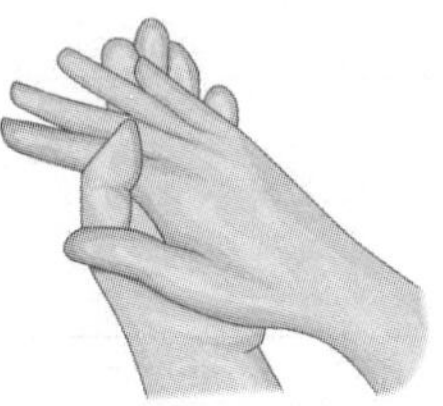

Palm to palm

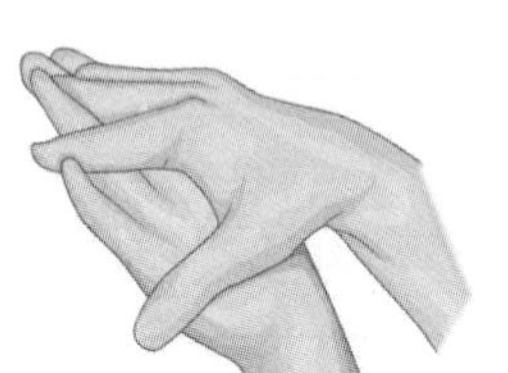

The back of one hands

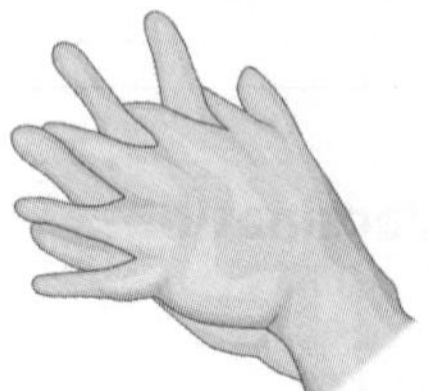

In between the fingers

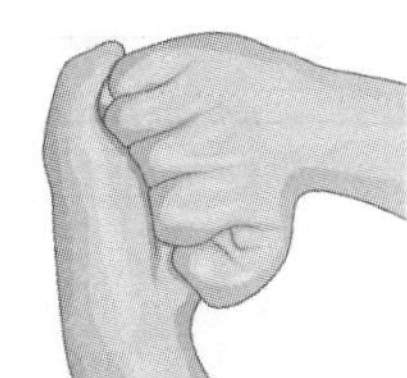

The back of the fingers

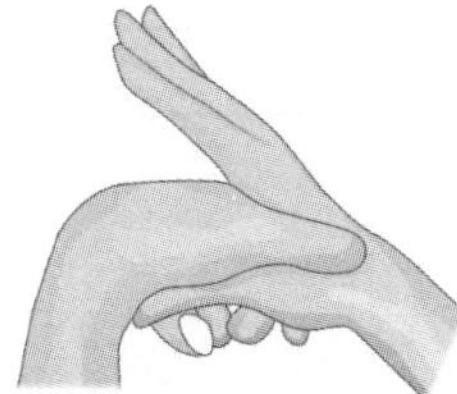

The thumbs

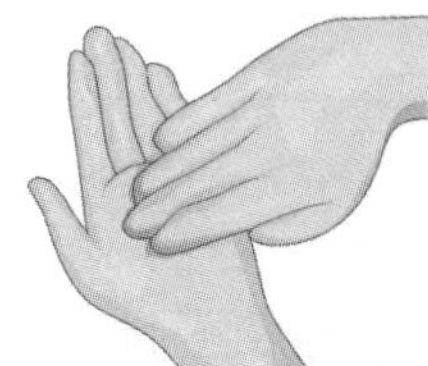

The tips of the fingers

Signature of the Academic Counselor/Supervisor

18.1: Oral Polio Programme Report

Name of the center: ____

Date and time: ____

Introduction

____
____
____
____
____

Objectives of Oral Polio Programme

____
____
____
____
____

Number of Participant in Programme

____
____
____
____
____

Method of Caring Vaccination

____
____
____
____
____

Transport Area

Arrangement of Places

Procedure

Records and Report of Oral Polio Programme

Conclusion

Signature of the Student

Date:

Signature of the HOD of Community Health Nursing

Date:

Signature of the Supervisor

Date:

18.2: Anemia Programme Report

Name of the center: ____

Date and time: ____

Introduction

____
____
____
____
____

Objectives of Anemia Programme

____
____
____
____
____

Number of Participant in Programme

____
____
____
____
____

Using Method of Awareness Programme and AV Aids

____
____
____
____
____

Report of Programmes and Conclusion

____
____
____
____
____

Signature of the Student   **Signature of the Supervisor**

Date: **Date:**

Signature of the HOD of Community Health Nursing

Date:

18.3: Vitamin A Deficiency Programme Report

Name of the center: ____

Date and time: ____

Introduction

____
____
____
____
____
____
____

Objectives of Vitamin A Deficiency Programme

____
____
____
____
____
____
____

Number of Participant in Programme

____
____
____
____
____
____

Using Method of Awareness Programme

____
____
____
____
____
____

Diet Plan of Vitamin A

Health Education of Vitamin A Deficiency

____
____
____
____
____
____
____

Conclusion

____
____
____
____
____
____

Signature of the Student

Date:

Signature of the HOD of Community Health Nursing

Date:

Signature of the Supervisor

Date:

18.4: Diarrhea Control Programme Report

Name of the center: ____

Date and time: ____

Introduction

____
____
____
____
____

Objectives of Diarrhea Control Programme

____
____
____
____
____

Number of Participant in Programme

____
____
____
____
____

Using Method of Awareness Programme

____
____
____
____
____

Methods Preparation of ORS (Home Preparation and ORS Pack)

____
____
____
____
____

Health Education of Diarrhea Control Programme

____

____

____

____

____

Conclusion

____

____

____

____

____

Signature of the Student

Date:

Signature of the HOD of Community Health Nursing

Date:

Signature of the Supervisor

Date:

18.5: Worm Infestation Control Programme Report

Name of the center: ____

Date and time: ____

Introduction

____
____
____
____
____

Objectives of Warm Infestation Control Programme

____
____
____
____
____

Number of Participant in Programme

____
____
____
____
____

Using Method of Awareness Programme

____
____
____
____
____

Health Education of Warm Infestation Control Programme

____
____
____
____
____

Conclusion

____
____
____
____
____

Signature of the Student   **Signature of the Supervisor**

Date: **Date:**

Signature of the HOD of Community Health Nursing

Date

18.6: Mental Health Programme Report

Name of the center: ____

Date and time: ____

Introduction

Objectives of Mental Health Programme

Number of Participant in Programme

Using Method of Awareness Programme

Conclusion

Signature of the Student　　　　　　　　　　**Signature of the Supervisor**

Date:　　　　　　　　　　　　　　　　　　　　**Date:**

Signature of the HOD of Community Health Nursing

Date:

18.7: School Health Programme Report

Name of the center: ____

Date and time: ____

Introduction

____
____
____
____
____

Objectives of School Health Programme

____
____
____
____
____

Group of Participant in Programme

____
____
____
____
____

Steps in School Health Programme

____
____
____
____
____

Conclusion

____
____
____
____
____

Signature of the Student   **Signature of the Supervisor**

Date: **Date:**

Signature of the HOD of Community Health Nursing

Date: